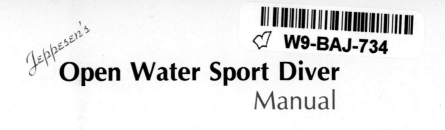

Jeppesen's

Open Water Sport Diver
Manual

Jeppesen's

Open Water Sport Diver
Manual

Richard A. Clinchy III, Editor
Emergency Medical Resources
Plantation, Florida

Glen Egstrom, PhD, Associate Editor
Underwater Kinesiology Laboratory
University of California, Los Angeles
Los Angeles, California

Lou Fead, Associate Editor
Author, *The Easy Diver*
Miami Shores, Florida

Fifth Edition

with 336 illustrations

Illustrations and artwork by Alan Thompson
Photography by Richard and Nancy Clinchy

A Mosby-Jeppesen Product

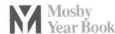

Mosby
Year Book

St. Louis Baltimore Boston Chicago London Philadelphia Sydney Toronto

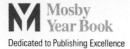
Mosby
Year Book
Dedicated to Publishing Excellence

Executive Editor: Richard A. Weimer
Developmental Editor: Rina Steinhauer
Project Supervisor: Lilliane Anstee
Design: Candace Fries

Photo credits: **Front Cover,** photograph by Ed Robinson/ Tom Stack & Associates.
Fig. 14-2, Bob Sheridan. **Fig. 14-3,** Bob Sheridan. **Fig. 14-7,** Jeff Bozanic.
Fig. 14-8, Jeff Stone. **Fig. 16-1,** Sandra Edwards.

A Mosby-Jeppesen Product

Fifth Edition

Mosby–Year Book, Inc.
11830 Westline Industrial Drive
St. Louis, Missouri 63146

Library of Congress Cataloging-in-Publication Data

Open water sport diver manual / Richard A. Clinchy, editor; Glen
    Egstrom, associate editor, Lou Fead, associate editor;
    illustrations and artwork by Alan Thompson; photography by Richard
    and Nancy Clinchy.—5th ed.
        p.   cm.
    Includes index.
    ISBN 0-8016-9035-8
    1. Diving, Submarine.   I. Clinchy, Richard A.   II. Egstrom, Glen
H.   III. Fead, Lou.
GV840.S78064   1992
797.2'3—dc20
                                                                        91-25040
                                                                        CIP

CL/SL/VH   9   8

Contributors

Gordon M. Boivin
Rescue Specialist, Canadian Coast Guard
Vancouver, British Columbia, Canada

Jeffrey Bozanic
Free-lance diver specializing in cave and
    cavern diving. Treasurer, NAUI
Los Angeles, California

Glen Egstrom, PhD
Underwater Kinesiology Laboratory
University of California
Los Angeles

Lou Fead
The Easy Diver
Miami Shores, Florida

William L. High
Founder, Professional Cylinder Inspectors
    Fisheries scientist, NOAA.
Seattle, Washington

Matt McDermott
Diving Safety Program, University of Cali-
    fornia, Santa Cruz
Santa Cruz, California

Milledge Murphey, PhD
Director, Academic Diving Program
University of Florida
Gainesville, Florida

Daniel Orr
Training Coordinator of Divers Alert Net-
    work (DAN)
Duke University Medical Center
Durham, North Carolina

Robert Rutledge, MD
Anesthesiologist and diving instructor
Owner, Training Ventures
Miami, Florida

Michael Steidley
Marketing Consultant with NAUI *and* Co-
    author, *Diving With Dive Computers*
San Diego, California

Acknowledgments

Completion of a book of this nature requires the contributions and cooperation of a very large number of people to make it an effort of which those of us coordinating the project can be proud.

I must thank the two principal people from Mosby–Year Book, Inc., who have been most involved in the completion of this book. Richard Weimer, Senior Editor, has provided immeasurable support, direction, and patient assistance in completing this project. Also, usually in Rick's absence, I have called upon Rina Steinhauer for her assistance and direction. They have both been there every time a snag has arisen and their help was needed.

To my Assistant Editors, Glen Egstrom and Lou Fead, my thanks for their lending their years of experience and wisdom to this project.

The contributors listed on p. v were confronted with a project of substantial proportions and impossible deadlines for their performance. All of them are major figures in the scuba diving field with full schedules of their own; each submitted their work on or before their assigned deadlines.

Much of the photography contained in the book was done in the Bahamas at the Peter Hughes Diving operation at the Divi Bahamas Beach Resort & Country Club, Nassau. My thanks to Peter Hughes and Craig J. Burns, Dive Operations Manager for Peter's operations, for his cooperation as well as the personnel at Divi Hotels for their assistance. Harry Ward, Manager of the Peter Hughs Diving operation in Nassau, was friendly, supportive, and made a mammoth shooting schedule go smoothly. Members of the Peter Hughes Diving staff deserving of special mention are Alan and Diana Roberts, Tony McKinney, Errol Lloyd, Andrew Higgs, Sean Lowe, and Wemzel Nichols.

Thanks go out to Bob and Marty Good, owners of Orbit Marine Sports, Pompano Beach, Florida, for their cooperation in completing many of the equipment shots.

Models who agreed to assist and who appear in this book and the Advanced Manual include Many Jane Lewis, Matt McDermott, Dalia Jakubauskas, Renee Roberts, Alan Roberts, Marty Knickle Good, Patrick McKinzey, Tony McKinney, Andrew Higgs, Sean Lowe, Wemzel Nichols, and many others who are not individually identifiable but who appear in group or distance shots.

Several manufacturers have been particularly cooperative in their assistance with this project. Of particular note are:

Ikelite Underwater Systems	**Oceanic USA**	**Submersible Systems, Inc.**
Indianapolis, Indiana	San Leandro, California	Huntington Beach, California

Finally, to my wife Nancy, no words would appropriately express my gratitude for her help. Throughout the completion of this project, she has been supportive in any way possible. She served as my principal model, was a sounding board for any major changes to the project, and helped me review hundreds of photographs. For her many contributions to this project she has my thanks and, as always, my love.

Richard A. Clinchy
July 1990

Reviewers, models, and others providing assistance for the Sport Diver project:

Divi Bahamas Beach Resort & Country Club, Nassau

Peter Hughes Diving, Nassau: Peter Hughes, Craig Burns, Harry Ward, Alan and Diana Roberts, Tony McKinney, Errol Lloyd, Andrew Higgs, Sean Lowe, and Wemzel Nichols

Orbit Marine Sports, Pompano Beach, Florida: Bob Good, Marty Knickle-Good, Patrick McKinzey, Mark Reamy

Divers Den, Ft. Lauderdale, Florida: Gary Smith, Dave Smalling, Bernardo Andrade

Samuel T. Scott, Arlington, Virginia

Paul Auerbach, MD, Vanderbilt University Medical Center, Nashville, Tennessee

William Cline, Dallas, Texas

Sharon Donovan, Moss Beach, California

Tom Griffiths, EdD, Pennsylvania State University, State College, Pennsylvania

Hammersmith International Inc., San Jose, California: Steven J. Hammersmith, Beth M. Hammersmith, Charles Chavtur, and Paul Allen Andersen

Jack Hezlep, Jeppesen Sanderson, Englewood, Colorado

Mary Jane Lewis, Dalia Jakubauskas, Stephanie Payne, Renee Roberts, Darrold Garrison, Diana DeNegre, Steve Hansen, Jeff Parker, Matt Stout, Seth Klein

Equipment manufacturers:

Ikelite Underwater Systems, Indianapolis, Indiana

Oceanic USA, San Leandro, California

Submersible Systems, Inc., Huntington Beach, California

Orca Industries, Inc., Toughkenamon, Pennsylvania

Force Fins, Santa Monica, California

Additional photography: Jeff Bozanic, Matt McDermott, Ikelite Underwater Systems

Contents

Introduction, 1

1 Seeing and Swimming, 3
MASK, FINS, AND SNORKEL, 4
Masks, 4
Fins and Footwear, 12
Snorkel, 20
USING THE MASK, FINS, AND SNORKEL TOGETHER, 23
Entries, 23
Surface Dives, 30
Ascending and Surfacing, 32

2 Warmth and Buoyancy, 33
Dive Skins, 34
Wet Suit, 34
Dry Suit, 41
Weight Belt, 42
Buoyancy Compensator, 46

3 Breathing Underwater, 51
Scuba Tanks, 54
The Regulator, 63
Buddy Breathing, 75
Buddy System, 78
Summary, 79

4 Underwater Information, 80
PRESSURE, TIME, AND DIRECTION DEVICES, 81
Submersible Pressure Gauge, 81
Underwater Timing Devices, 83
Depth Gauge, 84
Dive Computers, 86
Compass, 87
Natural Navigation, 90

5 Tools and Accessories, 92
SPECIAL EQUIPMENT AND TOOLS, 93
Float and Flag, 93
Whistle (Surface Signal), 94
Flare, 95

Dive Knife and Dive Tool, 95
Underwater Light, 96
Thermometer, 97
Logbook and Dive Tables, 97
Spare Parts and Repair Kit, 99
Gear Bag, 100
Summary, 100

6   **Sensations**, 101
FLOATING, SEEING, HEARING, AND EXPOSURE,   102
Floating, 102
Buoyancy, 102
Seeing, 104
Hearing and Speaking, 107
Hand Signals, 108
Exposure, 108
Summary, 115

7   **Breathing**, 116
RESPIRATION, PANIC AND EXHAUSTION, RESUSCITATION, CLEAN AIR,   117
The Respiration Process, 117
Gas Exchange, 120
Panic and Exhaustion, 123
First Aid for Drowning, 124
Cardiopulmonary Resuscitation (CPR), 125
Clean Air, 129
Summary, 130

8   **Descending and Ascending**, 131
Effects of Pressure Change, 132
Boyle's Law, 137
Squeezes, 138
Vertigo, 142
Decreasing Pressure, 142
Air Embolism, 142
Other Overpressure Injuries, 144
Prevention, 145
Summary, 149

9   **Depth and Time Limits**, 150
EFFECTS OF DIVING TOO DEEP AND TOO LONG, 151
Nitrogen Narcosis, 151
Oxygen Tolerance, 152
Partial Pressures, 152
Decompression Sickness,   153
Altitude Diving, 158
Flying after Diving, 159

Treatment of Decompression Sickness, 159
Summary, 160

10 Repetitive Dives, 161
RESIDUAL NITROGEN, MORE THAN ONE DIVE,
AND DECOMPRESSION DIVING, 162
Residual Nitrogen, 162
More Than One Dive, 162
Dive Profile, 164
Decompression Diving, 168
Aids to Dive Planning, 168
Summary, 170

11 The Worlds of Diving, 171
History of the Oceans, 172
Ecology, 173
Environmental Variation, 173
Weather, 176
Diving on the Water Planet, 178

12 Water Movement, 179
TIDES, CURRENTS, WAVES, AND THEIR EFFECTS
ON DIVING, 180
Tides, 180
Tidal Currents, 181
Ocean Currents, 183
Waves, 183
Localized Currents, 190

13 Ocean Life, 195
Reef Development, 196
Reef Inhabitants, 200
Dangerous Marine Animals, 205
Handling Marine Life, 207
Summary, 207

14 Fresh Water, 208
DIVING AREAS, 209
Lakes, 210
Rivers, 211
Sandpits and Quarries, 212
Natural Caves, 213
Sinkholes and Springs, 215
Mines, 215
Common Fresh-Water Animals, 215

15 Ecology, 218
Sources of Problems, 219
Coastal Problems, 221

Industry, 223
Sport Diving, 224
Inland Problems, 225
Solutions, 226
Summary, 226

16   Food from Sea and Lake, 227
Spearfishing, 228
Salt-Water Shellfish, 229
Fresh-Water Shellfish, 230
Salt-Water Crustaceans, 230
Commercial Development of the Seas for Food, 232

17   Dive Planning, 233
Conditioning, 234
Dive Objective, 236
Dive Site Selection, 236
Scouting the Site, 236
Equipment Preparation, 238
Environmental Considerations, 239
Weather Forecasting, 239
The Dive Day, 240
Predicting the Dive Conditions, 240
The Dive, 241
After the Dive, 242
Sport Diver Standards for Safe Diving, 243

18   Specialty Diving, 245
Cave Diving, 246
Cavern Diving, 250
Ice Diving, 251
Wreck Diving, 252
Treasure Hunting, 253
Blue-Water Diving, 254
Search and Rescue, 255

19   Careers, 256
Sport Diving, 257
Light Commercial Work, 259
Heavy Commercial Work, 260
Sciences, 260

Appendix, 262
Water Temperature Protection Chart, 262
Air Purity Standards, 263
Archimedes Principle and Gas Laws, 263
Air Consumption Formula/Table, 264
Sport Diver Open Water U.S. Navy Dive Tables, 265

Comparison of Several Popular Dive Tables, 265
Metric System, 269
Conversion Factors, 270
U.S. Weights and Measures, 271
Locating Your Nearest Recompression Chamber, 272
Equipment Check List, 273
First Aid Kit Components, 274

Introduction

This book, in its original form, was a product of Jeppesen Sanderson, Inc., a sister company of Mosby-Year Book, Inc.

The Jeppesen *Open Water Sport Diver Manual* was first published in 1975 and since then has been used by thousands of scuba instructors to train hundreds of thousands of people entering this wonderful world of scuba diving.

The original structure and content of the book have been left untouched where possible, but some sections have been slashed to remove material superfluous to the training of the open-water diver. All sections have been modified or rewritten to bring the material up to a level consistent with scuba as it exists in the last decade of the 20th century.

Robert A. Clark, the original principal author of this work, who has been anonymous over the years, did a magnificent job with the original work and much of it has been left alone.

This new *Open Water Sport Diver Manual* is to be used as part of an educational system developed to assist the instructor to teach scuba to the student: workbook, instructor guide, slides, and video tapes are all a part of what the system provides.

But all of these things cannot teach scuba skills to the student, and for that reason, the system leaves skill teaching and explanations largely to the individual instructor. The instructor must also structure the meaningful repetition of skills that will enable those skills to become second nature to the new diver.

This book and system are not meant to be a certification agency's system. Rather, the system is intended as an instructor's tool to teach scuba. Regardless of the agency for which you teach, this is a generic teaching tool which will fit any agency's standards.

We are confident that you will find *Open Water Sport Diver Manual* easy on the student and an effective teaching/learning tool.

1 Seeing and Swimming

- Mask
- Fins
- Snorkel
- Entries
- Surface Dives

OBJECTIVES

At the conclusion of Chapter 1, you will be able to:

1. List the main features of a dive mask.
2. Describe the difference between a low-volume and a wide-angle mask.
3. Properly fit a mask on yourself.
4. Describe how to equalize pressures within your mask.
5. Describe the difference between a full-foot and an open-heel fin.
6. Properly fit swim fins on yourself.
7. Identify two types of snorkel.
8. Describe how to clear a snorkel on a dive.
9. Describe when to use seated entries.
10. Describe when to use feet-first surface dives.

KEY TERMS

Refraction	Vented blade fin	Giant stride entry
Safety glass	Open-heel fin	Rigid snorkel
Equalization	Full-foot fin	Flexible snorkel
Purge valve	Scissors kick	Back-roll entry
Double skirt	Flutter kick	Seated entry
Defogging solution	Dolphin kick	Frog kick

Mask, Fins, and Snorkel

The basic equipment of the skin diver—the mask, fins, and snorkel—were developed to provide clear vision underwater, to increase the mobility of the swimmer, and to allow breathing with the mouth and nose submerged. The mask, fins, and snorkel are basic not only to skin diving, but also to scuba diving. They add so much to your ability to see, move, and breathe underwater that you will soon feel practically immobile without them.

This chapter will help you learn to appreciate the importance of good, comfortable, and reliable equipment. The best mask is the one that meets your needs, fits your face, and feels comfortable regardless of price. Likewise, there is no one type of fin or snorkel that is best for everyone or every diving environment.

MASKS

Remember the first time you opened your eyes under water? Everything was blurry, wasn't it? The human eye, though it sees well in air, does not work well in the water. The eye depends upon the bending of light rays (refraction) at the junction of the eye and air to focus an image on the retina. Not enough refraction occurs between the eye and water for focusing to occur. Surrounding the eyes with air was found to be the simplest solution for allowing proper focusing underwater. Early

Fig. 1-1 An early diver with tortoise-shell goggles.

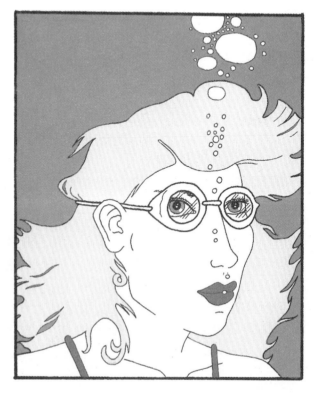

divers wore goggles with polished tortoise-shell lenses, similar to those pictured in Fig. 1-1. These lenses provided air spaces in front of the eyes to allow focusing and vision.

Swimming goggles are still available with tempered glass lenses and rubber straps, but these are not used by today's skin or scuba divers. Goggles can be used safely by surface swimmers to protect their eyes from chlorine and irritants, but, when the swimmer descends even a few feet, the increasing water pressure tends to squeeze the eyes into the air spaces in the goggles. This can cause eye injury even at shallow depths.

The first goggles solved the vision problem, but the pressure problem that they created was not solved until about 1865, when the first modern mask was invented. Instead of two small lenses with two airtight spaces, the modern mask has one large lens covering the eyes and nose in one common air space. (See Fig. 1-2.)

The single lens mask enables a diver to exhale through the nose and increase the air pressure within the mask to equal the pressure of the water outside the mask. With pressures inside and outside the mask the same, there is no squeezing of the mask against the face. The basic design of the early mask has remained essentially unchanged, but, as shown in Fig. 1-3, variations on the early mask add to the comfort, fit, and improved vision of the mask.

Fig. 1-2 *An early single-lens mask.*

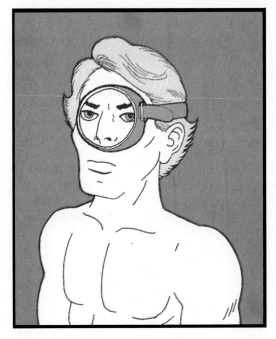

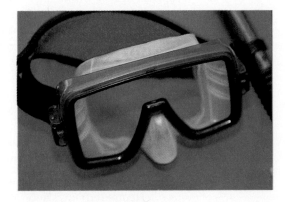

Fig. 1-3 *Low-volume diving mask.*

Selecting a Mask

The most significant improvement in mask design during recent years is the reduction in the mask volume.

Low-volume masks are designed to keep the air space inside the mask as small as possible. The lens fits close to your face and has a pocket for your nose. Many skin and scuba divers prefer this type of mask. With this type of mask it takes less exhaled air to clear water from inside the mask (a procedure explained later in this chapter) and to equalize pressure. (See Fig. 1-3.)

The wide-angle mask (Fig. 1-4) usually has a larger internal volume, which requires more air to clear the mask and equalize pressure than a low-volume mask. For this reason, it is more commonly used by scuba divers who have tank air to breathe than by skin divers, who only have the air in their lungs with which to clear and equalize. The wide-angle mask offers the addition of small glass plates on the sides of the mask which may enhance peripheral vision.

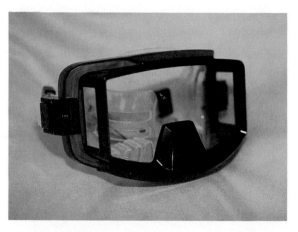

Fig. 1-4 *Wide-angle diving mask.*

Although masks are still available in rubber, a silicone compound is the most common material of which masks and mask straps are manufactured today. Silicone remains flexible throughout most temperature ranges and, when translucent, allows more light to filter into the mask than opaque materials do. Silicone is hypoallergenic, resistant to ozone deterioration, and requires only rinsing in clear fresh water and an occasional washing with mild soap. Rubber will remain relatively durable with proper care but may deteriorate as a result of exposure to heat, facial oils, and other environmental factors.

What to Look for in a Mask

As with any diving equipment, *fit and comfort* are the most significant considerations in the purchase of a mask. Once you have decided upon the type of mask you wish to own, look for the following features, which are illustrated in Fig. 1-5:

1. Make sure that the lens is tempered safety glass as indicated by the word "tempered" or "safety" printed directly on the lens. Tempered or safety glass will craze when broken rather than splintering.
2. The band surrounding the lens that holds it in place should be made of non-

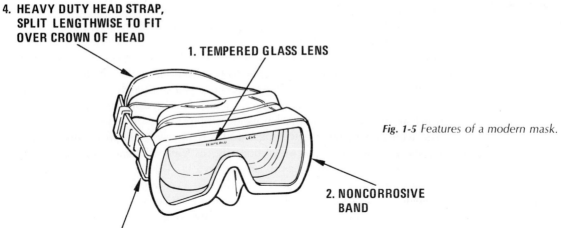

4. HEAVY DUTY HEAD STRAP, SPLIT LENGTHWISE TO FIT OVER CROWN OF HEAD

1. TEMPERED GLASS LENS

Fig. 1-5 Features of a modern mask.

2. NONCORROSIVE BAND

3. STRONG, EASILY-ADJUSTABLE BUCKLES WITH A POSITIVE LOCKING DEVICE

corrosive materials, such as hard plastic, for durability. It is removable to allow for replacement of a broken lens.

3. The strap should be split in the back for comfort and holding power. It should also be easily adjustable, have strong strap fastening buckles, with positive locking devices, and be easily adjustable for changes in diving environments and equipment.

A relatively recent innovation in mask straps is a wide one made of material similar to wet suit material. By using soft material and Velcro, it allows comfortable positioning of the mask without the hair pulling frequently associated with standard mask straps. (See Fig. 1-6.) Due to the comforts afforded by these straps and their ease of use, they are preferable over other mask straps available today.

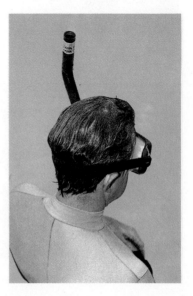

Fig. 1-6 The modern wide strap makes it easier to put on and take off your mask.

Mask Features

As you dive down under water, pressure around you increases. The pressure in the air spaces of your middle ears and sinuses must be equalized with the surrounding pressure to avoid injury. Some people can equalize by yawning or swallowing, while others exhale gently against a closed nose and glottis to equalize. Because of this, a mask may have a finger or nose pocket so you can pinch your nostrils shut in order to equalize; note Fig. 1-7. Equalization is discussed in detail in Chapter 8.

Masks do not stay perfectly dry inside while diving. A smile, laugh, or facial wrinkle can let water enter as the mask seal is temporarily released. Small amounts of water that leak in can be cleared easily, as you will learn. Some masks are equipped with a purge valve, as illustrated in Fig. 1-8, to assist you in removing water from the mask. The purge valve is a one-way valve that lets air and water flow out of the mask when you exhale, but does not let water flow into the mask. But if debris becomes caught in the purge valve, water can flow into the mask and make it impossible to fully clear the mask. It is for this reason that masks equipped with purge valves must be scrupulously cleaned after each use.

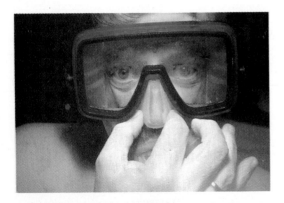

Fig. 1-7 Diver equalizing using nose pocket.

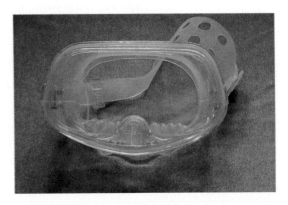

Fig. 1-8 Mask equipped with purge valve.

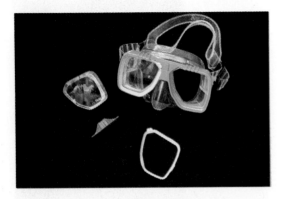

Fig. 1-9 Corrective lenses for diving masks.

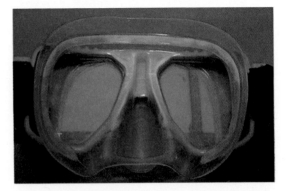

Fig. 1-10 The skirt of the mask should provide a double skirt against the face.

The diver who wears prescription glasses or contact lenses has several options for retaining corrected vision while diving. Some divers prefer masks with built-in corrective lenses. These are available through dive stores or optical companies that specialize in prescription diving masks. Fig. 1-9 shows masks with optical correction for use under water.

There is no reason why contact lenses cannot be worn while diving, if certain precautions are followed. As in any active sport, losing a lens is always a possibility, especially if a mask is suddenly flooded. Hard contact lenses are more easily displaced than soft lenses. The build-up and elimination of gas bubbles is another problem associated with contact lenses. Generally, gas-permeable lenses minimize that problem. If you wear contact lenses of any kind, *do not dive* until you have consulted an ophthalmologist knowledgeable in appropriate corrective lenses for diving.

To keep too much water from leaking into the mask, the skirt must form a good seal with your face. Most masks sold today use the double skirt shown in Fig. 1-10 to provide that good seal.

Mask Fit

One of the most important things about selecting your mask is finding one that fits the size and general shape of your face. The skirt of the mask should conform to the contours of your face without pinching or pressing harder in one place than another.

To make sure a mask fits properly, place it gently against your face without using the strap. The skirt should touch your face everywhere, with no apparent air leaks, gaps, or pressure points. Now, inhale gently, through your nose, with your mouth closed. This should pull the mask closer to your face without letting air leak in. If the mask fit is proper, the mask will stay in place while you are gently inhaling as described. See Fig. 1-11 for an example of testing mask fit. The mask should feel secure and comfortable. Try this test with several masks until you find one that is just right for you.

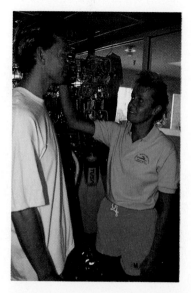

Fig. 1-11 Your dive store professional will assist you with mask fit.

Mask Use

A diving mask should have durable, easily adjustable strap fasteners attached to both sides. One way to don a mask is to put it in place on your face first, then slip the strap or straps over your head. (See Fig. 1-12.) Another way is just the opposite; put the strap on the back of your head first, then place the mask on your face.

The strap should be worn tightly enough to keep the mask firmly and comfortably in place. A loose mask strap will allow the mask to leak easily. If worn too tightly, the mask will squeeze uncomfortably against your face and cause leaks and headaches.

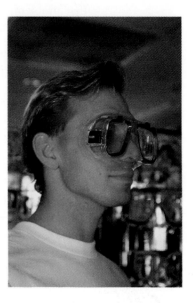

Fig. 1-12 Mask being put in place properly.

The strap should be placed on the head so that the pressure of the mask is applied evenly on the face. If there is too much pressure applied at the top or the bottom of the mask, it may leak. When putting your mask on or repositioning it under water, exhale gently through your nose to avoid the irritation of the water being forced into your nostrils as the mask is positioned.

The glass face plate of new masks is usually coated with a silicone protectant, which must be removed prior to use. If your mask comes with a gentle abrasive, clean both the inside and outside of the face plate with this material. If your mask does not come with cleanser of this sort, use nongel toothpaste or an instructor-recommended commercial mask cleanser for the same purpose.

A defogging solution, or some form of wetting solution, should be used on your mask prior to each dive. Without such an application, the warm humid air inside the mask will condense on the face plate as the glass contacts the cooler surrounding water in a dive. Defoggers will prevent the formation of droplets and fog on the face plate. Defoggers include commercially available chemical defoggers and liquid dishwashing detergents. With such defoggers, be careful to rinse the mask thoroughly after application so that your eyes will not be irritated by the chemicals. If the mask lens fogs over during a dive, let a little water inside your mask to rinse it clear.

One skill you will master in order to use a mask comfortably is mask clearing—removing all the water from the mask and replacing it with air while under water. This skill is easy, even when the mask is completely flooded. By pushing gently against the top portion of the mask against your forehead, tilting your head back and toward the surface, and exhaling through your nose, you create a greater pressure inside your mask than outside. By starting to exhale before tilting your head back, you may avoid unnecessary irritation of your nostrils by water trapped in the mask. This procedure forces the air and water out of the bottom of the mask or through the purge valve, as shown in Fig. 1-13.

When clearing a mask with a purge valve, the valve should be at the low point of the mask, to allow water to drain through it and is cleared by exhaling into the mask. Small purge valves are designed primarily for clearing the little bit of water that collects in the nose pocket.

If fully flooded, masks with small purge valves should be cleared the normal way. Masks can be cleared in almost any position as long as the highest part of the mask is firmly sealed against the face during exhalation. Fig. 1-14, for example, shows a diver clearing the mask from the side.

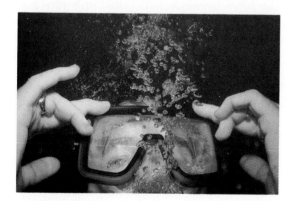

Fig. 1-13 Mask clearing.

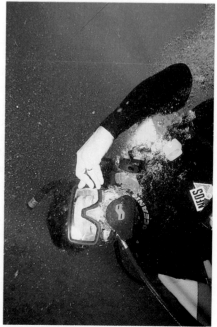

Fig. 1-14 Using basic principles of mask clearing, you can do it from any position.

As you descend, you should equalize the pressure inside the mask and inside your ears early and often. To equalize the mask, gently breathe air into it through your nose; otherwise, the increasing water pressure will tend to squeeze the mask against your face. A severe mask squeeze can cause small blood vessels in the whites of the eyes and the skin of your face to bleed. Mask squeeze is extremely uncommon in trained divers.

Ear squeeze, closely related to mask squeeze, is a more common diving problem. The following simple measures will help you dive without ear squeeze:

1. Always test to be sure you can equalize before you dive. You should be able to feel a slight pressure change in your ears when you gently exhale against a closed nose and glottis. Pinching your nose shut during a dive is done by using the nose pocket of your mask. Some people can equalize by swallowing, wiggling their jaws, or by using what is called the Frenzel maneuver, in which you exert pressure against the roof of your mouth by pressing with the tongue. Regardless of the method you use, just remember that the pressure you wish to create within the ears is a gentle pressure; do not blow too hard or you may injure your ears. This clearing process should be started immediately before you descend. Since the process of equalization involves air travelling up through the eustachian tubes into the middle ear, it is a good idea to "exercise" the eustachian tubes before an anticipated dive trip. For one or two days prior to your anticipated diving activities, clear your ears a few times each day to make sure that you will minimize the possibility of clearing difficulties on the day of the dive. This is simply another form of conditioning for your diving, and you may find the clearing is made easier if you practice ahead of time rather than waiting until the day of the dive to see if your ears are clearing adequately.

2. Do not dive with a cold even if you can equalize. Nasal congestion can worsen during a dive, making equalization difficult, and perhaps lead to ear injury.

3. Equalize before you feel ear discomfort. If discomfort does occur, STOP, ascend several feet above the point where the discomfort stops and then attempt to equalize.

4. If you cannot equalize, abort your dive. Do not permit any discomfort to persist during the dive.

5. Descend slowly and equalize often. A good rule of thumb during slow descents is to equalize with each exhaled breath or each foot of descent, whichever is more frequent.

For a closer look at equalization, see Chapter 8.

FINS AND FOOTWEAR

Under water, a good swimmer can move fairly well for short periods of time without special equipment. But prolonged swimming, even for a highly trained athlete, demands an extraordinary amount of strength and endurance.

With the advent of rubber foot fins in the 1930s, underwater swimmers gained increased mobility and efficiency without expenditure of extraordinary effort. Fins substantially increase the surface area of the naked foot and enable greater thrust forces to be developed. They enable the diver to swim greater distances for longer periods of time without tiring.

Selecting Fins

Fins fall into two general categories: the full-foot fin and the open-heel fin as shown in Fig. 1-15. Full-foot fins are built much like the rubber shoes you may have had as a youngster for rainy days except that there is a blade attached to each. They come in different sizes similar to normal shoe sizes. Open-heel fins usually come in four different sizes: small, medium, large, and extra large. The strap of the open-heel fin is used for limited size adjustment for fit.

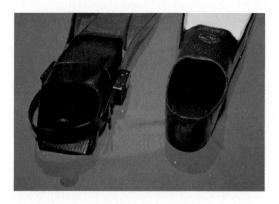

Fig. 1-15 Full-foot and open-heel fins.

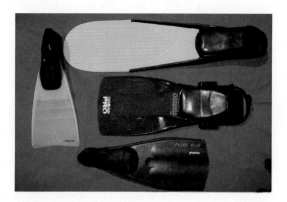

Fig. 1-16 Fins come in a variety of blade lengths and types.

What to Look for in Fins

As in selecting a proper mask, it is necessary to know what features to look for when choosing the right fins for your diving activities. The essential considerations are discussed below.

Purpose. Fins should be selected with diver size, leg strength, and diving conditions in mind (Fig. 1-16). An open-heeled fin provides for the option of using booties for cold water or rocky shore diving, and some size adjustment. If you will usually be diving from a boat in warm water, the full-foot fin may be your best choice. If, however, you will be diving in a variety of environments and will be using booties for some of your diving but not for all, the open-heel fin should be your choice. Blade length and stiffness will be a matter of leg strength (comfort) and expected diving conditions, such as significant currents (safety).

Materials. Notice the quality of the material and manner of construction. Fin blade material may be black rubber, graphite, polyurethane, thermoplastic, or a composite material. All types are durable and provide good service when cared for properly. Generally, the stiffer the blade and the longer the fin, the more power the fin can develop. However, more leg strength will be needed to drive the stiffer fin. "Space-age" materials such as graphite, thermoplastics, and polyurethane are not as susceptible to ultraviolet and ozone deterioration as is black rubber. Thermoplastic blades may warp if exposed to high temperatures. Fin pockets are usually made of softer material for enhanced foot comfort.

Buoyancy. Fin material also determines the buoyancy of fins. Some fins sink, some float, and others are neutrally buoyant (neither sink nor float). Although less important than blade size, stiffness, fit, and comfort, fin buoyancy may be considered in selection. If you plan to dive in relatively deep water with limited visibility (not recommended for the beginning diver), fins that float might be better since you won't lose them as easily. When diving in clear, shallow water, it might be easier to keep track of fins that sink.

Fit. Open-heel fins have the advantage of fitting better than fins that are not adjustable. A fin that is too tight can restrict circulation and cause foot cramps, while fins that are too loose can rub, chafe, fall off, or cause cramps from muscular efforts to keep the fin on.

Blade Design. Vented-blade fins, illustrated in Fig. 1-17, *A* and *B*, have several slots, or vents, located along the blade to redirect the flow of water through and along the fin. This is purported to provide less tiring leg strokes and give maximum power. Other modified blades are designed to cup water flow for a powerful downstroke and split it for an easier upstroke. Fig. 1-17 also shows a rather unusual fin design, which has become particularly popular with snorkelers, that employs design concepts that are certainly unique and not in keeping with classic fin design.

To gain maximal thrust from your fins, you should probably seek fins which are long, narrow, and as stiff as your leg strength will tolerate. If possible, you should try several fin varieties for comfort, fit, power, and efficiency in the water before you commit to purchasing a particular fin.

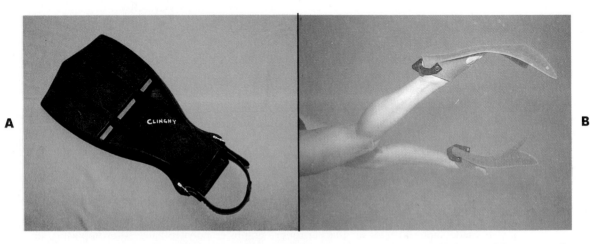

Fig. 1-17 A, The vented blade fin. *B,* A unique fin design, which utilizes different muscles than conventional fins and generates propulsion power in a different manner.

Fin Fit

Selecting fins to fit properly over booties depends on the size of the foot pocket and the strap. (See Fig. 1-18.) Booties are made of wet suit material and are necessary for foot protection, and added warmth when diving in cold water. Many divers prefer booties for warm water diving as well to protect their feet when walking on rough surfaces to a dive site. The foam material of the booties serves as a cushion between the foot and the fin pocket, minimizing the possibility of blisters. Tennis shoes or socks are poor substitutes for boots and should not be used as a replacement for proper footwear. They do not protect against cramps and cold, and they do not stop sand and other debris from causing blisters. Booties cushion the foot against the stresses of foot pockets which may not perfectly match the anatomical shape of the diver's foot but are designed to fit the diver's booted foot.

When selecting open heel fins, try them on over a pair of wet suit boots. Adjust the straps so the fins are firmly in place, and try to kick them off. They should remain in place and feel secure without binding, cramping, or pinching.

Full foot fins should fit comfortably over bare feet, should not bind or be too tight, and should be shaken in the same manner as the open heel fin to assure they remain securely on the foot (Fig. 1-19).

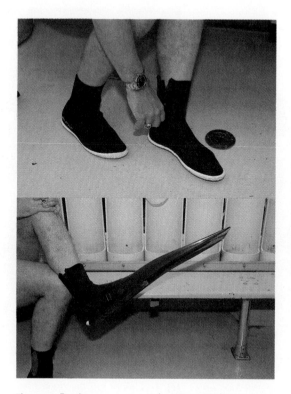

Fig. 1-18 *Putting on wet suit bootie and trying open-heel fin for fit.*

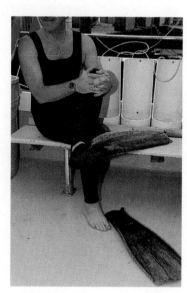

Fig. 1-19 *Trying full-foot fins for fit.*

Fin Use

There are a few tricks to putting fins on your feet. Most divers put on their fins dry, but when diving from something *other* than a boat you should wet your feet, booties, and fins so the fins will slip on more easily. If you are using full-foot fins, fold the heel back to form a "handle" to pull on. With open-heel fins, work the fin pocket over the foot as far as possible and then slip the strap over the heel instead of pulling the fin on by the strap. Figs. 1-20 and 1-21 illustrate the donning of both types of fin.

Few things feel as clumsy as trying to walk wearing fins on your feet. In fact, walking forward while wearing fins can be rather dangerous. (See Fig. 1-22.) Walking backward, when necessary, on the beach or in shallow water is much easier and safer, if you watch where you are going. For safety reasons, walking in your fins in other settings, especially boat decks and pool decks, should be avoided.

Climbing boat or pool ladders while wearing fins is usually not recommended, though there are some boat ladders specifically designed to allow divers to climb safely while wearing fins. An easier approach to climbing ladders is to remove the fins while still in the water, hold them in your hand, or slip the straps over your

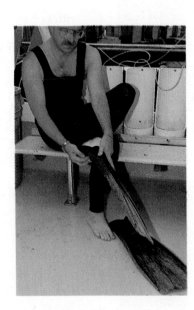

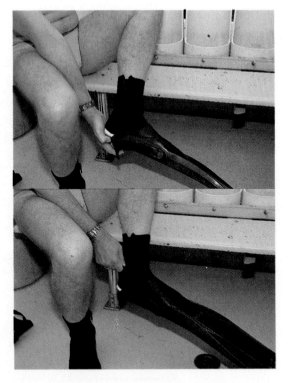

Fig. 1-20 Donning the full-foot fin by folding the foot pocket underneath to use as a "handle."

Fig. 1-21 Donning the open-heel fin by slipping the foot into the foot pocket first, then pulling the fin strap over the heel.

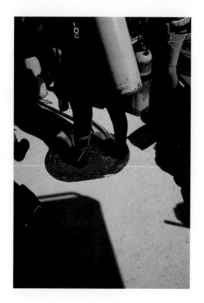

Fig. 1-22 For reasons of safety and to prevent injury to yourself, you should never wear your fins on a dive boat or on a pool deck as this diver is doing.

wrist, then climb the ladder. Do not lose positive connection with the boat when your fins are off because without fins you have little capability of moving purposefully while wearing a scuba tank.

If water conditions permit, and there is no current that might sweep you away from your diving boat should you slip off the ladder, you may prefer to lay your fins on the diving platform or deck of the boat or hand them up before climbing aboard. From a safety standpoint, it is best to keep your fins with you until you are on the boat.

When you enter the water, fins become powerful extensions of your own body. In fact, fins are so effective that your arms and hands are not necessary for propulsion when skin or scuba diving. Instead, you can let your arms trail alongside, or use your hands for changing directions, exploring, or carrying equipment or treasures. One note of caution has to do with touching things while in the water: please avoid touching anything that looks as though it is or might be alive. In the salt water realm, tremendous coral damage is done by contact from divers' fins and hands, and the more conscientious you become about this from the very beginning of your scuba diving adventure, the better and more responsible diver you will be. Unnecessarily stirring up the bottom deposits sand on coral colonies and thrashing the bottom with fins tends to impair visibility.

Kicking

The flutter kick, pictured in Fig. 1-23, is the most widely used kick in diving. It is a slow, wide, and steady kick that moves a lot of water with each stroke. Knees flex naturally to direct energy to the rear and ankles swing back and forth like hinges. There is no reason to swim fast—doubling your speed in water takes four times the effort. When doing the flutter kick at the surface, be sure to keep your legs and fins well under the water by raising your head a bit.

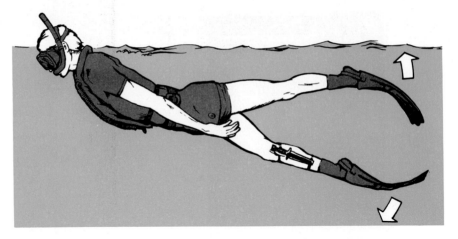

***Fig. 1-23** Flutter kick.*

The scissors kick is sometimes used to let tired flutter kick muscles relax. The first stroke is almost identical to the flutter kick but with little power applied. Notice the similarity in Fig. 1-24. The power stroke, bringing the legs together, stops when your feet come close to each other. After gliding for two or three seconds, repeat the first stroke with the same leg coming forward and the same one going back. Because of the glide feature in the scissors kick, it is more relaxing and restful than a speed kick.

The frog kick is not commonly used in diving, but is good for providing a restful variation in kicks on long surface swims. Occasionally changing to the frog kick, for example, puts different muscles to work than those used in either the flutter or scissors kick. As a result, your legs will not tire as easily and will be less likely to cramp. The frog kick begins with a slow separation of your legs, as shown in Fig. 1-25. The power stroke brings your legs together forcefully and ends in a long easy glide which lasts until you lose most of your forward momentum.

The dolphin kick is a useful variation underwater. As seen in Fig. 1-26, both legs stay and work together. Begin the dolphin kick in a horizontal position. Bring your fins up by bending your legs at the knees; then, bring your legs down in a power stroke by straightening your legs and bending slightly forward at the waist. The next step is to bring your fins up again by bending at the knees slightly and, at the same time, straightening your body at the waist and arching your back. As you gain speed, your body moves forward in a wave-like motion that starts at your head and travels along your body as it does for a dolphin or whale.

Since the dolphin kick has both fins working together instead of balancing each other, it is the kick that works best with only one fin and is therefore quite useful if you lose a fin while diving.

Another resting variation for surface swims is swimming on your back. You can keep your direction constant by using a compass or keeping some stationary objects in line, with an occasional look toward your objective to confirm your course.

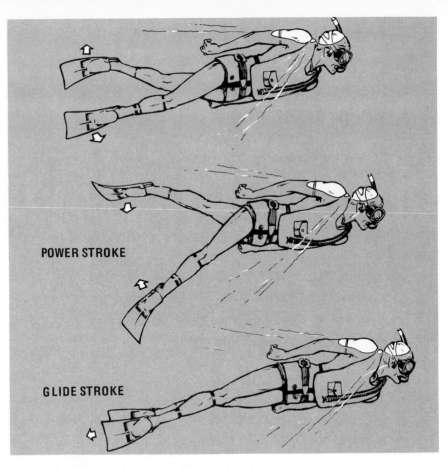

POWER STROKE

GLIDE STROKE

Fig. 1-24 *The steps in the scissors kick.*

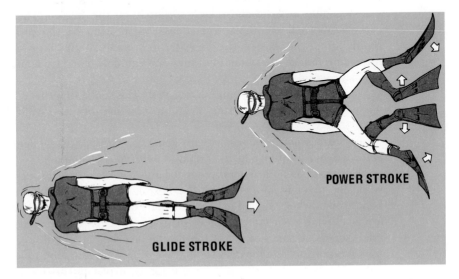

POWER STROKE

GLIDE STROKE

Fig. 1-25 *The frog kick.*

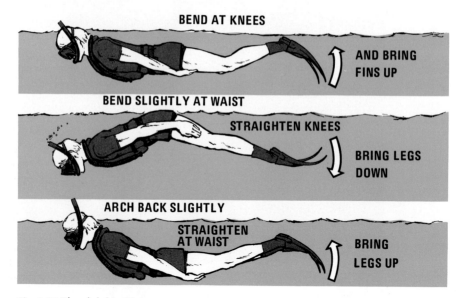

Fig. 1-26 *The dolphin kick.*

SNORKEL

Breathing tubes of one kind or another have probably been used for over 2,000 years, but it was not until the snorkel joined with the modern mask and fins that man was able to swim and relax effortlessly on the surface. The snorkel, with its curved tube and mouthpiece, enables you to swim on the surface without constantly lifting your face above the water to breathe. With your head down and body relaxed, you have maximum buoyancy and can float along for hours viewing the underwater world.

The snorkel is also a scuba diving tool. The scuba diver uses it to conserve air while swimming on the surface, to and from a dive site, and while surveying a dive area.

For discussion purposes, we are going to establish two general classes of snorkel: rigid and flexible. Fig. 1-27 shows both types of snorkels.

The rigid snorkel generally has a large internal bore for easy breathing even when the diver is finning hard. The flexible snorkel is made of material that will bend or flex when tangled or snagged, for example, in kelp. In general, unless you are in a diving environment where snags are anticipated, there is no need for a flexible snorkel. A modification of the flexible snorkel is the "drop-away" snorkel that uses a corrugated segment of tubing which permits the mouthpiece to drop easily out of the way when the scuba regulator is in place. This has become a popular snorkel type with many scuba divers.

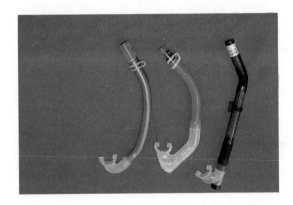

Fig. 1-27 Rigid and flexible snorkels.

What to Look for in a Snorkel

Two major factors to consider when selecting a snorkel are breathing resistance and comfort. A snorkel that has a large bore and clean, simple lines with gentle curves is usually easy to breathe through.

A snorkel does not have to be long to work well. Excessive length, in fact, increases breathing resistance and rebreathing of exhaled air. Breathing resistance also is increased when the snorkel has sharp curves, a reduction in bore size, or corrugations inside the snorkel tube. For some divers, a barrel with an excessively large bore can be difficult to clear of water.

Some snorkels have a one-way purge valve or self-draining valve near the mouthpiece for easy clearing. (See Fig. 1-28.) When you surface, the water in the upper part of the tube above the surface drains out through the submerged valve by gravity flow. The remaining water can be blown out with a short, forceful exhalation to fully clear the snorkel.

Since a snorkel mouthpiece that does not fit can be extremely uncomfortable, be sure to test it for fit in your mouth when selecting it for use. Mouthpieces are available in many different sizes, shapes, textures, degrees of flexibility, and materials. Most modern snorkels allow you to adjust the position of the mouthpiece for

Fig. 1-28 Snorkel purge valve.

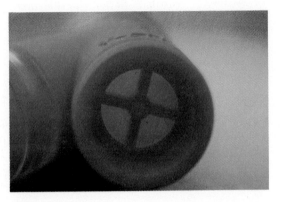

comfort. Some can even be molded to the precise imprint of your teeth for added comfort. Silicone materials are the best for mouthpieces, since they tend to be the most comfortable and are hypoallergenic, should you be sensitive to synthetic materials. Try several different snorkels until you find one that feels comfortable and allows you to breathe easily.

Snorkel Use

As shown in Fig. 1-29, the snorkel is normally worn on the left side to avoid confusion with the scuba regulator hose and second stage, which are on the right side. The snorkel is attached to the mask strap with the help of a device created for that purpose. Some masks are supplied with rigid attachment systems; there are Velcro-based attachment systems for the snorkel, and the longest-standing method is the snorkel-keeper, sometimes called a butterfly.

The snorkel-keeper is a double-ring device made of rubber or silicone. One ring is first slipped over the snorkel barrel, then the keeper is placed around the mask strap, and the other ring is slipped over the snorkel barrel. Once the snorkel is attached to the mask strap, its position in the snorkel-keeper is adjusted until the mouthpiece feels comfortable; the snorkel will be nearly vertical when you are swimming on the surface with your face under the water, looking down at a 45-degree angle.

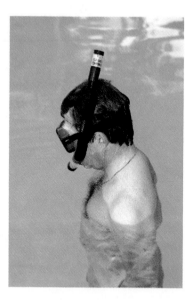

Fig. 1-29 Appropriate snorkel placement.

When you dive below the surface, the air in the snorkel will bubble out through the top and water will fill the snorkel barrel. There are two different ways to get rid of this water when you return to the surface. The most common method is to blow hard and fast into the snorkel, as shown in Fig. 1-30. This is called "popping" or "blasting" the snorkel clear, because the water is popped or blasted up and out of the tube very quickly. Be careful not to blow around the mouthpiece. After clearing the snorkel, your first breath should be slow and shallow to keep from inhaling any water that may remain in the snorkel. Sometimes a second, less forceful blast of air will clear any remaining water in the snorkel.

When swimming at the surface, it is not uncommon for water to spill into the snorkel. When it does, simply blast it clear. This soon becomes second nature and you will automatically clear your snorkel regularly.

The expansion or displacement method of snorkel clearing is used when returning to the surface. As you ascend, lift your face to look toward the surface. This points your snorkel parallel to the surface or slightly down. (See Fig. 1-31.) As you approach the surface, exhale lightly into your snorkel. The gentle exhalation clears the snorkel easily as the end of the snorkel tube clears the water. This method is easier than blasting the snorkel clear, but it works only if your face is lifted upward as you break the surface.

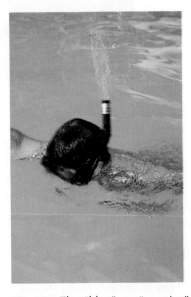

Fig. 1-30 *The "blast" or "popping" method is the way to clear a snorkel without adjusting head position on the ascent.*

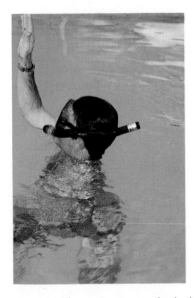

Fig. 1-31 *The expansion method of snorkel clearing.*

Using the Mask, Fins, and Snorkel Together
ENTRIES

Entry into the water should be easy, safe, and not disorienting. It should be a transition, not a collision. The entry should leave diving equipment in place and ready to use. It should leave you oriented to which way is up and which way is down. Finally, regardless of the type of entry, it is desirable to be positively buoyant prior

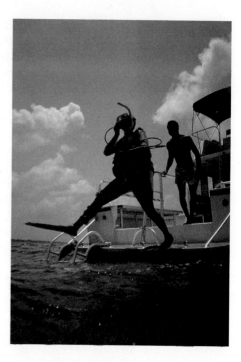

Fig. 1-32 The giant stride entry.

to entry.* If you are properly weighted when diving, you should be neutrally buoyant at the surface and not require any air in your buoyancy compensator to remain neutrally buoyant. Some surf entries and exits may actually be made more dangerous if an inflated buoyancy compensator is used.

Before every dive, evaluate your entry area and the dive site. Make sure the water is deep enough for the entry and there are no hidden hazards. You should also be aware of any currents in the area.

Before entering, perform a final "buddy" check to make sure both of you are ready to enter. If you are entering first, make sure your buddy knows that. On all entries, grip your mask with one hand as you enter. Once in the water, return to the surface, turn to face your entry point and signal your dive buddy or the dive master that you are okay, then move out of the entry area. Watch while your buddy enters so you can assist, if needed.

Boat, Dock, and Pool Deck Entries

Feet-first entries generally work well when you are entering from a firm surface such as a large boat, dock, or pool deck. They keep you in an upright position so you can maintain orientation throughout the entry. Fig. 1-32 shows the most popular feet-first entry, the giant stride being made from a boat diving platform. The idea of the giant stride is to step into the water with your legs spread, and then forcefully kick your legs together following entry to stop your downward progress and keep your head above the surface.

---

*The buoyancy compensator, discussed in detail in Chapter 2, should be one third to one half full of air for most scuba entries. For such diving entries, the buoyancy compensator should be about half full.

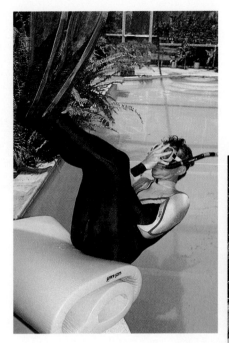

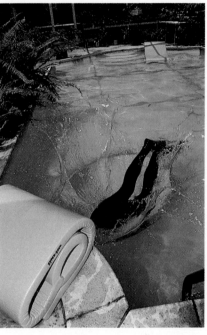

Fig. 1-33 *The back roll entry.*

Other types of feet-first entries are the walking and jumping entries. The walking entry is for entering from surfaces essentially at the same level as the surface of the water. The diver simply walks into the water while holding the face mask in place.

The jumping entry is more appropriate for entering from surfaces over 6 feet above the water.

The back roll entry, shown in Fig. 1-33, is used most often for diving from a small boat or rubber raft when standing, to do a giant stride, might be unsafe. Two divers should back roll off a raft at the same time to keep it from rocking. The back-roll entry can leave you slightly disoriented in the water.

In still water another entry is made by lowering your tank with attached buoyancy compensator inflated into the water to don it there on the surface. Being properly weighted is a must for this technique to prevent you from sinking before donning your gear. Figs. 1-34 through 1-38 illustrate donning scuba gear in the water.

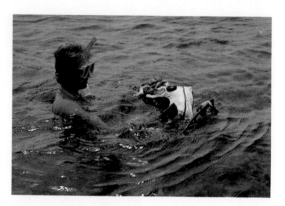

Fig. 1-34 Gear into the water with buoyancy compensator partly inflated and diver properly weighted.

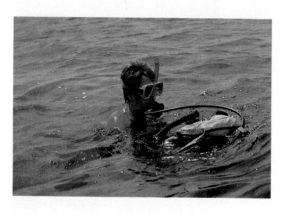

Fig. 1-35 Second stage regulator is placed in the diver's mouth and the buoyancy compensator is drawn toward the diver's right shoulder.

Fig. 1-36 Right arm is placed through the right side of the buoyancy compensator.

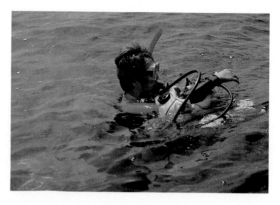

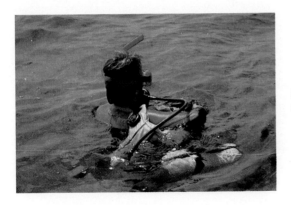

Fig. 1-37 Buoyancy compensator and tank are moved into position.

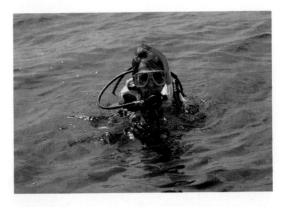

Fig. 1-38 Equipment in place and receiving final adjustments.

This entry is also used by divers who fear that lifting their gear might cause injury to their backs or who simply lack the strength to lift scuba gear into place for diving. For these divers, a buddy would lift the gear into the water.

The controlled seated entry is excellent for use from a low pool deck or boat platform. Simply sit on the deck or platform with your feet in the water, put all your gear on, put your regulator in your mouth, then turn and slip gently into the water, as shown in Figs. 1-39 through 1-44. This entry is completely controlled because you stay in contact with the boat or pool deck at all times, have little impact with the water, and remain oriented and in full control throughout.

Shore Entries

When making an entry from a shore, have your mask on, your regulator or snorkel in your mouth, and weight belt, tank, and buoyancy compensator in place. You will have to decide whether or not to wear your fins. If you have to climb over rocks or through mud, it is probably safer and easier to carry your fins into the water until it is deep enough for you to float; then, put on your fins and swim out to dive.

Ocean beach entries through the surf breaking near shore usually include donning fins on shore, then shuffling backward until in water deep enough to turn around and swim out through the surf. If the surf is breaking far out from the shore, you may carry your fins out to knee-deep water and put them on out there. (See Fig. 1-45.)

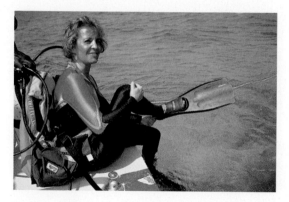

Fig. 1-39 *The fins and other gear are put on while comfortably aboard the dive boat or while sitting on pool deck.*

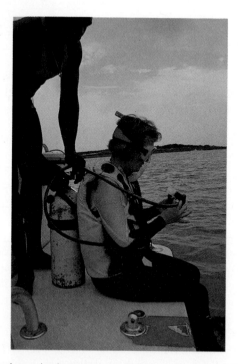

Fig. 1-40 *With mask in place, the buoyancy compensator is put on with assistance from the dive master. Before preparing to enter the water, the regulator goes in the mouth and all equipment is in place.*

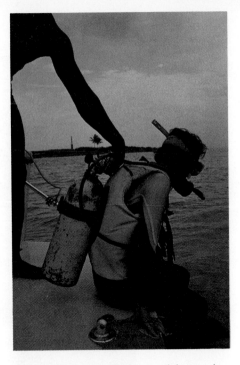

Fig. 1-41 The controlled, graceful entry begins.

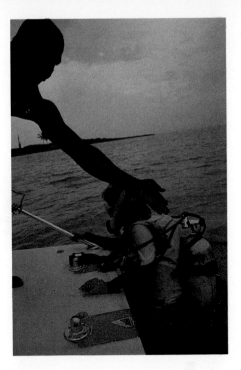

Fig. 1-42 The diver turns to face the platform.

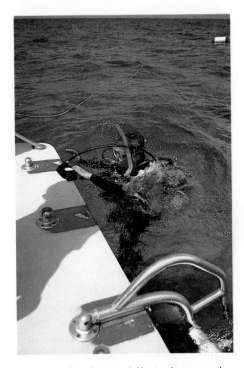

Fig. 1-43 The diver is fully in the water but still in contact with the platform.

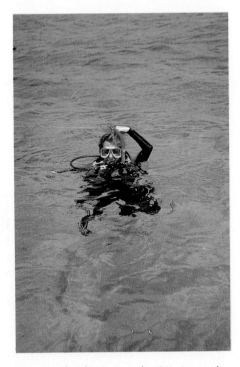

Fig. 1-44 The diver gives the OK sign to the buddy, dive master, or boat.

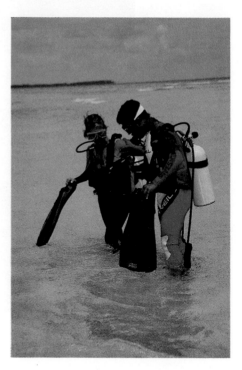

Fig. 1-45 *Entering from shore may require either putting on fins before entering or carrying your fins.*

Remember, do not try to walk forward in the water with fins on your feet. Realize also that shuffling will help you maintain your balance while "kicking-out" any rays that might be buried in the sand. More information concerning beach entries is given in Chapter 12 and under "Beach Diving" in the *Advanced Sport Diver Manual*.

SURFACE DIVES

Whether skin diving or scuba diving, it is recommended that you be with a buddy. While skin diving, divers usually take turns for diving or for observing from the surface so you always know what your buddy is doing.

There are two basic types of surface dives: the head-first and feet-first. The purpose of both types is to initially lift part of your body out of the water so its weight can then push you down into the water. If done properly, the head-first dive can take you 8 to 20 feet below the surface without kicking.

The head-first surface dive, pictured in Fig. 1-46, starts from the face-down floating or swimming position with your legs near the surface. First, bend your body at the waist to force the top half of your body straight down. Then lift your legs up completely out of the water. This is the key to the head-first surface dive. If you get your legs out of the water straight over you, they will create the greatest downward force to take you down easily.

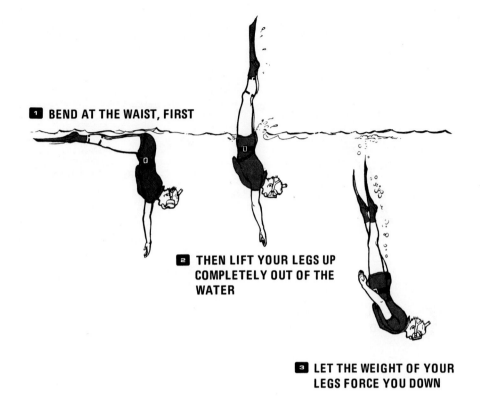

1 BEND AT THE WAIST, FIRST

2 THEN LIFT YOUR LEGS UP COMPLETELY OUT OF THE WATER

3 LET THE WEIGHT OF YOUR LEGS FORCE YOU DOWN

Fig. 1-46 *The steps in the head-first surface dive.*

In order for the properly weighted scuba diver to descend, it should simply be a matter of breath control.* The properly weighted diver will sink below the surface when he or she fully exhales.

The feet-first surface dive is used primarily by divers in kelp where there is not enough room to swim or float horizontally at the surface and is also useful for limited visibility entries. It lets you begin in a floating, vertical position. (See Fig. 1-47.) The objective is to lift your upper body as far out of the water as possible, to provide the downward force for your dive. Start by separating your legs in a flutter-kick position and putting your arms on the surface. Then kick hard and bring your arms down quickly. As you lift up and out of the water, keep your arms against your sides, then drop straight down beneath the surface. When below the surface, stroke your arms up to help force you down. When you stop descending, tuck yourself into a ball, turn your head down, and swim toward the bottom. As stated previ-

---

*A diver is neutrally buoyant when in the vertical position; the diver remains at or just below eye level with about one half breath in the lungs.

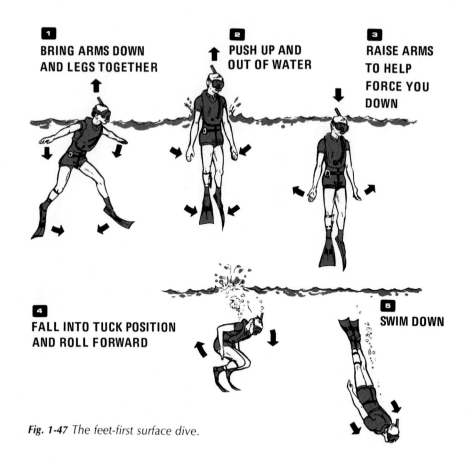

1 BRING ARMS DOWN AND LEGS TOGETHER

2 PUSH UP AND OUT OF WATER

3 RAISE ARMS TO HELP FORCE YOU DOWN

4 FALL INTO TUCK POSITION AND ROLL FORWARD

5 SWIM DOWN

Fig. 1-47 *The feet-first surface dive.*

ously, however, the properly weighted scuba diver should be able to slowly descend simply by exhaling.

ASCENDING AND SURFACING

As you ascend to the surface to end a skin dive, extend your arm as protection from obstructions above and to point to the surface. Look up and turn so you can see boats or other objects which may be in your path. Upon surfacing, clear your snorkel, leave your mask in place, and breathe through your snorkel with your head and face in the water. Relax and take advantage of your natural buoyancy.

Buoyancy can be increased by keeping your lungs full between breaths. If you intend to stay on the surface for some time, inflate your buoyancy control device. Throughout your ascent and rest at the surface, you should always be aware of your buddy's location and condition.

Scuba diving ascents are different in that air supply allows a more leisurely ascent; you can change your ascent rate or descend to avoid surface obstacles. Concerns for avoiding decompression sickness or air gas embolization may require control of ascent speed and timing. This is discussed in greater detail in Chapter 8.

2 Warmth and Buoyancy

- Dive Skins
- Wet Suit
- Dry Suit
- Weight Belt
- Buoyancy Compensator

OBJECTIVES

At the conclusion of Chapter 2, you will be able to:

1. Name three types of protective garments worn by divers.
2. List three types of thermal protection for divers.
3. Explain the method by which wet suits keep the diver warm.
4. Name three features that may be found in wet suits.
5. Describe the steps in donning a wet suit including pants, jacket, and hood.
6. Explain how to care for your wet suit following a dive.
7. State how to evaluate whether you are neutrally buoyant.
8. Name two types of weight belts.
9. Name the type of buoyancy compensation device appropriate for snorkeling.
10. Name three features you should look for in a buoyancy compensator.

KEY TERMS

Dive skin	Neoprene	Ditching
Wet suit	Lycra	Inflator
Dry suit	Variable-volume	CO_2 cartridge
Farmer Johns	Booties	Horse collar
Buoyancy compensator		

Modern diving equipment solved the problems of seeing and swimming underwater but did not solve the new problem of cold. Prolonging diving time when wearing just basic skin diving equipment causes a diver to feel the discomfort of cold.

Other diving mammals such as whales and otters have protective blubber or thick, oily fur to insulate them, whereas divers must wear protective suits to retain body heat. The protective suits of choice range from thin Lycra dive skins and foam-neoprene wet suits to variable-volume dry suits.

DIVE SKINS

The thin Lycra dive skin allows divers in warm water to have some minimal thermal protection and provides protection from abrasive coral and barnacles (Fig. 2-1). "Skins," as they are called, are currently available in an endless variety of color combinations and may even be impregnated with ultrathin neoprene to add an extra amount of thermal protection for those extended warmer water dives.

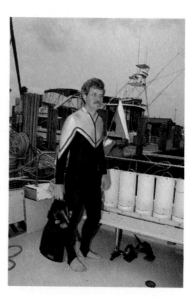

Fig. 2-1 *The typical, popular Lycra or composite dive "skin."*

Skins also provide a number of other benefits. They can be worn under other exposure protection for additional thermal benefit and to facilitate donning the other protection. Colorful dive skins also add an exciting dimension to underwater photography.

WET SUIT

Since water absorbs body heat 25 times faster than air, a temperature that might be uncomfortably warm in air could become uncomfortably cold in water. A resting diver, for example, chills in about 1 hour when the water temperature is between 75° and 80° F (approximately 25° C). Cold water, however, is not only uncomfortable, but also is dangerous. People have died within 1 hour in 40° F (4° to 5° C) water.

During the first attempts to solve the problem of cold, divers wore long underwear covered with a waterproof rubber dry suit. The smallest leak or tear in the dry suit, however, ruined everything; divers quickly found soggy underwear and thin rubber suits to be poor insulators.

Divers also discovered that they did not have to be bone dry to stay warm. Preventing body heat from escaping simply required an insulating material to prevent it from passing into the water. A wet suit made of foam neoprene, ³⁄₁₆- to ¼-inch thick, does that.

Foam neoprene is synthetic rubber filled with tiny bubbles. It is widely believed that the wet suit warms the body by allowing a thin layer of water to enter between the neoprene and the skin, which is then warmed and actually insulates the body. However, this is not altogether desirable, because if there is room for the water to enter in the first place, there is room for water to circulate. If the water circulates, it must be continually rewarmed, which pulls body heat away. It is better to have a suit that fits snugly enough to stop all water circulation into, inside, or out of the suit. No water circulation lets you stay warmer than even very little circulation.

Wet suit material thicker than ¼ inch provides increased insulation but also increases buoyancy and tends to restrict movement. Whatever the thickness, as a diver descends, increased pressure compresses the material. Consequently, its buoyancy and insulation are diminished.

Diving comfort is greatly increased by a good wet suit. This is especially true in water temperatures below 75° F (24° C), where much sport diving takes place. In many areas, a wet suit extends the diving season from a few summer months to all year. A wet suit also protects against the sun and almost anything else that could irritate, bruise, chafe, or harm delicate human skin. The wet suit also provides extra buoyancy which can be used in an emergency.

Selecting a Wet Suit

Sport divers commonly dive in water between 40° and 75° F (4° to 24° C). In this temperature range most divers find it best to cover the entire body with a wet suit, including hood, gloves, and boots.

In warm water, you may need only a ⅛-inch thick jacket. In cooler water, a hooded vest and shoulder-high pants, sometimes referred to as "Farmer Johns," may be added to help keep your torso warm. Figs. 2-2 through 2-4 show three types of wet suit protection. It is important to remember that hypothermia may also occur in warm water due to long exposure without adequate protection.

The extent of body coverage and thickness of necessary wet suit protection depend on many things. Thin divers, for example, need more protection than overweight divers. Extremely active divers need less protection because they produce more body heat. All divers generally need extra protection when diving in deeper, colder water, especially in fresh waters below the thermocline.

When you are selecting a wet suit, the water temperature you plan to dive in is a primary factor to consider. Your choice of suits includes both standard sizes and

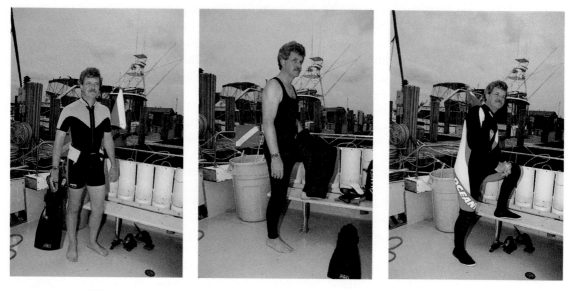

2-2   2-3   2-4

Fig. 2-2 *The "shortie" provides minimal wet suit protection with the trunk primarily being protected.*

Fig. 2-3 *The design of the "Farmer Johns" provides an extra layer of thermal protection to the trunk.*

Fig. 2-4 *This wet suit is of one piece and is a choice favored by many divers who require full wet suit protection but feel they are more comfortable than they would be in a two-piece garment.*

custom-made suits. The correct fit is best for maintaining warmth and allowing comfortable movement. A suit that is too tight can keep you warm, but it restricts breathing, circulation, and freedom of movement. Custom-made suits ensure a perfect fit, but stock sizes are acceptable if they fit snugly and feel comfortable.

What to Look for in a Wet Suit

After deciding on the type of wet suit protection you need, study the neoprene material and see how it is made. Wet suits lined inside and out with four-way stretch fabric are the most durable. The inside lining makes it easier to climb into; it works like a dry lubricant. The external lining slightly reduces the flexibility of the suit, but increases its strength and suit life. Suits without nylon, or with nylon on one side, are equally warm but are difficult to put on and take off without a dry powder lubricant.

Wet Suit Features

Zippers at the ankles and wrists make dressing and undressing easier but may not be necessary. Usually an extra strip of neoprene is put under zippers to restrict water leakage. If you plan to dive in extremely cold water, avoid wet suits with zippers unless you must have them for fit or dressing purposes.

Wet suit jackets are available with a spine pad, which is an extra strip of foam neoprene that fits into the depression along your spine. The spine pad restricts cold water from circulating in this space. Pockets, reinforcing patches, knee and elbow pads, and special knife or tool holders also can be built into wet suits.

Special pockets may be built inside wet suits that permit the insertion of reusable, chemically activated hot packs, which add extra warmth to the body, particularly at the base of the spine or at the chest, in extremely cold environments.

Neoprene boots are available with soft soles for swimming comfort, or with tough rubber soles to protect both boots and feet when walking over sharp rocks or coral.

The one wet suit feature that is not optional is good fit. A suit should feel snug all over your body without binding or pinching. There should be no significant gaps or spaces under the arms, at the neck, or in the crotch. The ankles, waist, wrist, and neck openings should be tight enough to keep water from sloshing in and out, but not tight enough to reduce circulation. In short, your wet suit should fit like a second skin.

Wet Suit Use

Using a wet suit is easy. Once you have it on, you can forget about it and enjoy its warmth. Getting it on and taking it off is the challenging part. Dressing can be frustrating, time consuming, and exhausting the first few times, or when the suit is too tight. Some divers wear either nylon or Lycra undergarments (e.g., dive skins) to make dressing easier. Another trick developed to ease the donning and removal of wet suits is to place baby shampoo diluted to approximately one-half strength into a spray-pump bottle and spray your body immediately before putting the suit on. The dilute baby shampoo makes your body "slick" and eases the donning of the suit.

To avoid any confusion, follow these steps when preparing for entry on your first dive, especially when you do not own the equipment. Normally, all equipment is tried on for proper fit and adjusted prior to leaving for the dive site. It is important to remember to begin dressing only after an evaluation of the dive site and dive planning activities are completed.

1. **Pants.** Pants go on first (Fig. 2-5). Fold the pants down over the knees as though you were turning them inside out, then pull them on over your feet. This ensures a good fit from the ankle to the knee. Once the pants are on up to the knees, simply roll them up your legs, checking that the crotch fits snugly. To prevent overheating during dressing, it may be advisable to don one piece of the suit at a time, pausing between suit parts to cool yourself off if necessary. Wet the remaining parts of the suit as you do so to remain comfortable.

2. **Boots.** If using boots not equipped with zippers, roll the top of the boots down and inside out (Fig. 2-6). Then work the foot into the boot as far as you can before pulling it over your heel and ankle. Nylon diver's socks greatly

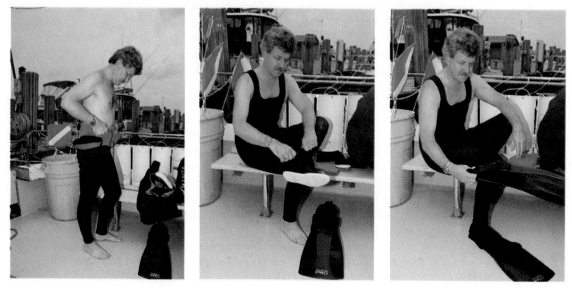

2-5   2-6   2-7

Fig. 2-5 Donning wet suit pants.

Fig. 2-6 Wet suit boots with zippers make donning them somewhat easier.

Fig. 2-7 Checking fins for proper adjustment.

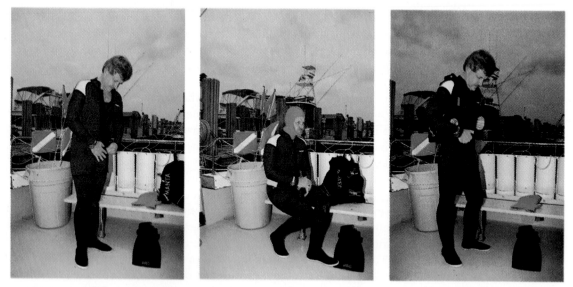

2-8   2-9   2-10

Fig. 2-8 Donning the wet suit jacket.

Fig. 2-9 Donning the wet suit hood.

Fig. 2-10 The BC is donned over the wet suit jacket to check for proper fit and comfort.

assist in taking boots on and off. Zippers in pant legs are useful to help tuck the boot tops under the wet suit pants. Tucking helps keep sand out of the boots on a beach entry. Zippers in the boots greatly ease donning the boots with the tops tucked inside the pants in the same manner. A ballooning effect often occurs when water draining from the interior of the suit is forced into the boot after the dive if the boot top is over the wet suit ankle seal. If the boot is under the ankle seal of the suit, water drains out over the exterior of the boot.

3. **Fins.** Put the fins on over your boots to check for proper adjustments (Fig. 2-7). Then, lay them near the staging area so they will be handy when you prepare for your entry. Have all the equipment you need in the staging area before putting on the rest of your wet suit. On warm days, you can become overheated if you delay entry while wearing a wet suit.

4. **Jacket.** Pull the wet suit jacket on like any ordinary shirt or jacket, one arm at a time (Fig. 2-8). If the jacket has a step-in design, legs must go in first. Pull the sleeves up all the way to your armpits so there are no gaps under your arms. When they are not up all the way, they will pull and bind your shoulder and create discomfort and limit arm movement. Before zipping the jacket, fasten the crotch strap, if necessary, to help hold the flaps together.

5. **Hood.** Put the hood on next (Fig. 2-9). Pull it from the front of your forehead down and toward the back of your head so it will pull your hair out of the way. The lower skirt of the hood should be tucked under the collar of the wet suit jacket if it has a cold water skirt. Otherwise, it may be worn outside the jacket.

6. **Buoyancy compensator (BC).** If using a horse-collar BC, adjust the waist and crotch straps so that they are snug when it is fully inflated (Fig. 2-10). Jacket-style or low-profile BCs do not necessarily need special preparation, as adjustments can be made once they are on. It is a good idea, especially when using rental equipment, to don your BC over your wet suit to check for fit, comfort, and ease of movement with the BC inflated.

7. **Weight belt.** The weight belt goes on after any BC that uses a crotch strap (Fig. 2-11). For most jacket-style BC/tank combinations that do not employ a crotch strap, it is much easier and safer to put the weight belt on before the BC. Placing it on after the tank drastically complicates the dressing process, especially on a rocking boat.

  The weight belt should be put on in such a way that other equipment will not interfere with its removal. Make sure that the weights are positioned slightly forward of the hips to prevent the weights from shifting during the dive.

  No more than 6 inches of webbing should extend beyond the buckle once the appropriate number of weights are on the belt. Excess webbing may be cut off and the material treated to prevent unraveling. Excess webbing should *never* simply hang down. If the rental or borrowed weight belt has excess strap extending well beyond the buckle, the buckle should be moved, webbing cut, or the belt exchanged for another, rather than being tucked in or secured in any fashion that could restrict emergency removal.

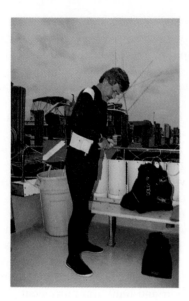

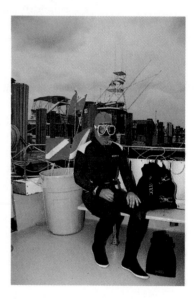

Fig. 2-11 *The weight belt is next properly put on with particular attention being paid to the ability to remove the weight belt without interference from any other equipment.*

Fig. 2-12 *Mask in place with mask seal against face and not interfered with by hood material.*

In order to promote consistency in dealing with emergencies, the diving community generally recommends that the buckle be placed in such a way as to allow for release with both hands. Regardless of the recommendation, divers are cautioned to include buckle familiarization as part of their predive preparation.

8. **Mask.** Put the mask on to make sure it is adjusted properly (Fig. 2-12). The mask skirt should be seated firmly against your face *underneath* the hood. After adjusting both mask and snorkel, lay them next to your other equipment.

9. **Gloves.** Gloves are the last piece of the wet suit to put on. Gloves go on like ordinary gloves, but must be pulled on completely. A glove only half on is clumsy and tiring. Your buddy can help in tucking the gloves under your sleeves at the wrist in the same manner the boots are tucked under your pant legs. Some cold water gloves are worn on the outside of the wrist seal because of the gauntlet-style design.

Wet Suit Care and Maintenance

After the dive, remove your equipment and wet suit, reversing the order in which you put it on. Rinse the wet suit inside and out in clear, fresh water. Hang it on wide wooden or plastic hangers in an open, shaded area to dry. You may even want to consider the purchase of special hangers, which are made especially for dive gear. Wet suit shampoo is now available from several manufacturers.

For permanent storage, do not fold the suit. Folds and creases in neoprene compress and weaken the material. Excessive heat and direct sunlight are also harmful.

Use neoprene cement to mend small tears. Lubricate metal fittings and zippers with silicone, candle wax, or even a bar of soap to keep them working smoothly. Occasionally, wash the wet suit with a mild detergent in lukewarm water. Many divers use the bathtub for washing and the shower head for rinsing. Open all snaps, zippers, and Velcro closures and slosh the suit up and down in the tub water for at least 5 minutes.

DRY SUIT

Dry suits, as the name implies, are designed to keep the diver dry (Fig. 2-13). This is accomplished by neck and wrist seals, a waterproof zipper, and attached boots. The suits work on the concept that air insulation is better insulation than water to keep a diver warm. Dry suits are, therefore, recommended for diving in extremely cold water or for extended bottom times in moderately cold water.

Dry suits are generally of two basic types: the foam neoprene, similar in design to a wet suit; and the shell design made of a shell of thin outer materials, including crushed foam neoprene, coated rubber, nylon pack cloth, vinyl or composite laminated materials, coupled with an insulating undergarment to keep the diver warm.

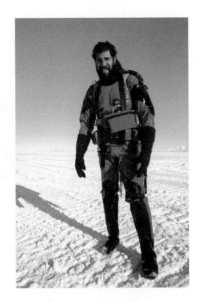

Fig. 2-13 *This dry suit and gear are used for especially cold water exposure.*

The type and thickness of the undergarment depend on the water temperature and anticipated workload, and some other minor factors.

To counteract the effects of pressure on the layer of air insulation surrounding the diver, dry suits have inflator/deflator systems similar in design to those found on buoyancy compensators. Even though the suit provides some buoyancy compensating capability, a BC should always be worn and used, since the suit air may escape inadvertently through a seal. Because of the complicated nature of the dry suit system, new divers are cautioned to gain considerable open water experience or specific dry suit training before selecting and using this type of exposure protection. A dry suit specialty course is suggested for all divers before using a dry suit in the open water.

WEIGHT BELT

Most divers in the water wearing a full wet suit or a dry suit float very well. The diver will be warm and comfortable but, without a weight belt to counteract the excess buoyancy of the suit, will be trapped at the surface. A lead weight belt is the solution to this buoyancy problem. Start with the selection of the appropriate amount of weight so that the BC can be used only for buoyancy corrections caused by compression of the suit at depth. The BC is, therefore, not to be used as a substitute for errors in proper weighting. Do not use a BC to compensate for too much weight on your weight belt.

Selecting a Weight Belt (Suggested Approach)

How heavy should a weight belt be? Each diver must experiment to find an answer. Your goal is to be neutrally buoyant at the surface (Fig. 2-14). To conduct this experiment, prepare your weight belt with an initial weight load and several

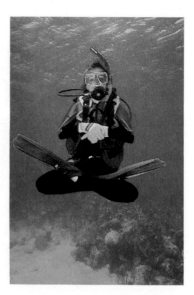

Fig. 2-14 *Achieving neutral buoyancy is the ultimate objective that you are seeking when selecting appropriate weight.*

pounds of clip-on weights. In cold water, diving with a ¼-inch wet suit, one way to estimate your initial weight load would be to start with approximately 15 percent of your body weight plus 5 pounds. When diving in climates that require less exposure suit protection or in fresh water, which is less buoyant, seek local guidance (or your instructor's advice) since a variety of wet suit thicknesses and different types of hoods and vests are used in these conditions.

To determine the exact amount of weight necessary, put on all the equipment you normally wear during a dive. Partially inflate your buoyancy compensator and enter calm water with your dive buddy, dive master, or instructor assisting you. Move to a depth where you can stand with your head clear of the surface and begin to adjust your weight as you slowly release air from your buoyancy compensator. You have achieved neutral buoyancy when, with your buoyancy control device completely deflated, you are floating at eye level with your lungs partially full. You should sink slightly when you exhale and rise slightly when you fully inhale.

As you descend, the effects of pressure will cause your wet suit to compress, and it will lose buoyancy. Some weight belts have an elastic compensator or a compensating spring buckle which constricts the weight belt, maintaining proper fit as the diver descends.

Neutral buoyancy is maintained at depth by using the buoyancy control device. Buoyancy is affected by the type, thickness and size of the exposure suit, tank material and pressure, the diver's body, the depth of the dive, and the density of the water.

Some aluminum tanks start out at 1 pound negative and can become as much as 4 pounds positive at the end of the dive as they near 500 psi. Do not adjust your weight belt for positive buoyancy at the surface before a dive. To do so may result in difficulty controlling your ascent as you approach within 15 feet of the surface. It is particularly important to control your ascent, especially during the last 20 feet of your dive. Being positively buoyant before a dive is not safe and may lead to an uncontrolled ascent near the surface. Positive buoyancy is properly established at the surface by using your buoyancy control device.

Weight needs are different for each individual diver and they often change. Remember to establish neutral buoyancy at the surface before beginning any dive.

Whether you choose to be neutrally buoyant at the surface or at depth, never wear more weight than necessary.

Since you are somewhat more buoyant in salt water than in fresh, remember to add between 2 and 5 pounds of lead when going from fresh to salt water. These are only general guidelines. Weight needs are individual and often change depending on the age and condition of the suit, equipment type, and quantity of exposure protection worn. A change from a full suit to a shortie or dive skins would result in a significant reduction in the amount of weight needed for the dive.

What to Look for in a Weight Belt

Fig. 2-15 shows the typical weight belt made of nylon web because it is strong and durable. Some weight belts include rubber segments that make the belt self-compensating for changes in belt length needed, depending upon depth as wet suit material compresses.

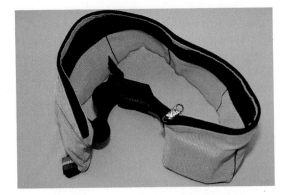

Fig. 2-15 *One of the types of weight belts available for divers.*

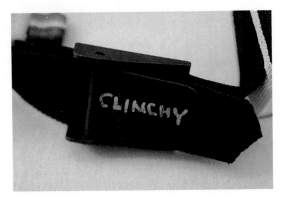

Fig. 2-16 *The quick-release buckle for the weight belt must be easy to release with either gloved hand and easily distinguishable on the diver.*

When pressure increases, the gas in the foam neoprene or the air in the dry suit is compressed, making the suit thinner and reducing the insulation and buoyancy.

Some weight belts contain pouches for solid lead weights or pouches containing lead shot.

The weight belt must be easily distinguishable from other equipment buckles and be a quick-release type as shown in Fig. 2-16. You should be able to release it immediately with both gloved hands. The clasp-type quick-release buckle may have a prominent notch to help reduce confusion with other buckles. The wire buckle is useful because it is unlike any other scuba equipment buckle and, therefore, prevents confusion with the buoyancy compensator or backpack buckles. The wire buckle, however, makes weight correction and adjustment more difficult.

There are different sizes of lead weights, as shown in Fig. 2-17. Some have slits so they can be donned or taken off without unbuckling the belt. Hip weights are

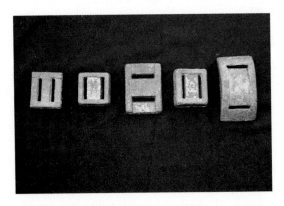

Fig. 2-17 *Lead weights come in a variety of sizes with the hip weights in 6 or 10 pounds.*

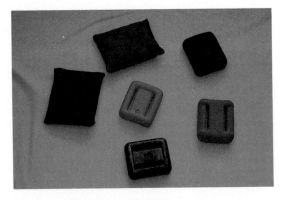

Fig. 2-18 *In addition to lead weights and lead weights covered with vinyl, there are weights that are actually shot-filled pouches.*

available in many weight designations and should be used as pairs and worn to balance each other. Some weights are vinyl coated to help protect boat and pool decks. Vinyl-coated weights are available in a variety of colors.

The shot-filled weight belt or belt composed of individual shot-filled pouches does not use ordinary lead weights (see Fig. 2-18). It uses shot—a mass of tiny lead balls—contained in a vinyl compartment. Shot is added or removed to adjust for differences in buoyancy. This is more complicated than changing lead weights and the vinyl compartment is more bulky; yet it is a more comfortable belt because the shot conforms to the body.

Using the Weight Belt

The exposure suit–weight belt combination is a dynamic safety pair. It protects you from the hazardous effects of cold and helps you to achieve instant buoyancy in an emergency. The weight belt helps you approach neutral buoyancy yet gives you positive buoyancy the instant you take it off in response to an emergency. This positive buoyancy at depth does not shoot you to the surface, but it does make it easier for you to swim up faster. To have this instant flotation available, the weight belt must not be held in place by other straps or equipment.

A quick-release buckle enables you to ditch the belt immediately. Simply unfastening the buckle is not enough, though. You must pull the belt completely away from your waist as far as you can so you can see it drop freely and clearly, as shown in Fig. 2-19; otherwise, it could get hung up on other straps, a knife handle, or even a fin. Frequent practice of this critical skill on land will assure its proper use during an emergency situation.

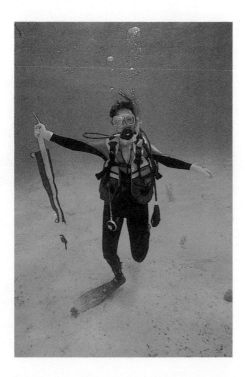

Fig. 2-19 In ditching the weight belt, the belt must be held well away from the body before it is released.

Your weight belt allows you to achieve positive buoyancy the instant you release it in response to an emergency. The amount of buoyancy will be directly related to several factors including the depth of the dive, but the strongest effects are how much exposure protection you are wearing and the amount of air in your BCD. A ¼-inch wet suit will offer much more buoyancy than a warm water ⅛-inch shortie.

In an emergency, anything that impedes your ascent to the surface, such as full collecting bags, artifacts, or salvage, should be dropped. After all, nothing you collect during a dive can possibly be worth your life. In an emergency, the procedure "Stop, Breathe Easy, Think, and Act" should be followed. If it becomes necessary to drop your weight belt, then perform the act deliberately and be prepared to control your ascent to the surface. Ditching the weight belt when you do not have free access to the surface may not help you in an emergency, since you will be positively buoyant when you contact an overhead obstruction and you may be trapped against it.

BUOYANCY COMPENSATOR

At this point, the complete buoyancy control problem has not yet been solved. The weight belt adequately counteracts the buoyancy of the suit at the surface, but buoyancy changes when you descend because of suit compression. If a medium-size wet suit has 18 pounds of buoyancy at the surface, for example, it may have less than half that buoyancy at a depth of 100 feet. The diver who wears 18 pounds of lead to achieve neutral buoyancy at the surface may find himself as much as 10 pounds negative at 100 feet. The buoyancy compensator (BC) was designed to help you counteract changes in buoyancy.

Selecting a Buoyancy Compensator

There is a wide variety of buoyancy compensators. The one shown in Fig. 2-20 is commonly referred to as a "horse collar" BC designed primarily as a floating device

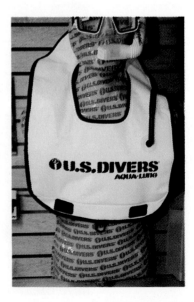

Fig. 2-20 *The horse-collar BC was the original BC used in diving and is now the BC used today in skin diving.*

for downed pilots or shipwrecked sailors. They were the original buoyancy compensators used for diving and still are the ones primarily used by skin divers. A necessary feature is an oral inflation/deflation tube to manually increase or decrease the volume of air inside the BC. Skin diving BCs also may be equipped with a CO_2 inflation device that can be activated to achieve positive buoyancy quickly once during a dive. A skin diving BC may be equipped with an overexpansion relief valve that automatically releases air when the BC is overinflated. The "horse collar" is no longer recommended as the buoyancy compensation device for scuba.

The low-profile BC, shown in Fig. 2-21, is designed specifically for scuba diving. Most of the buoyancy available is located around the waist and under the arms to provide lift at the surface, since the lifting air remains underwater. During a dive, the buoyancy is located around your natural center of gravity near the weight belt. A wide cummerbund helps reduce the tendency for the BC to ride up. Adjustable shoulder straps allow a comfortable fit and make it easier to put on or take off. Like all BCs used for scuba, it is equipped with an overexpansion relief valve and an oral inflation/deflation tube. Almost all BCs have a connector for a low pressure power inflator which allows you to inflate the compensator with air directly from the scuba tank. A dump valve also is included on most buoyancy compensators to allow air to be rapidly released for descent or to control your rate of ascent. The valve can normally be activated by a lever, pulling a string, or pulling the inflator hose.

The buoyancy control jacket shown in Fig. 2-22 is another buoyancy compensator for scuba diving. It has a large internal volume with the buoyancy located around the waist and over the shoulders. This buoyancy control jacket normally is equipped with the same features as the low-profile BC.

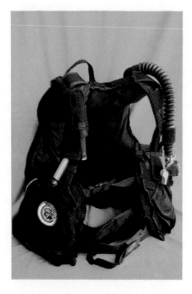

Fig. 2-21 *A low profile BC is popular among scuba divers.*

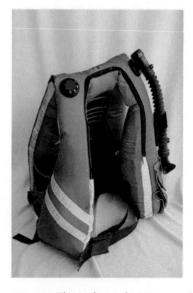

Fig. 2-22 *The jacket-style BC is another of the common scuba buoyancy compensators.*

Some compensators may have a modified scuba regulator for emergency breathing included in the power inflator feature. This usually allows the diver to breathe air from the scuba tank, not from the buoyancy compensator itself.

A buoyancy control pack is another alternative. It is usually a horseshoe-shaped unit that is attached to the tank backpack. This configuration places the buoyancy behind you, which removes some of the straps and bulkiness in front and makes it easy to rest or snorkel in a horizontal position either face down or face up. Some manufacturers have included a system of weights in the pack.

What to Look for in a Buoyancy Compensator

The construction of the BC usually falls into one of two broad categories—double bag or bladderless. The double bag design has an inner bladder protected by a strong fabric shell. In the single bag design, the shell itself serves as the bladder and is usually referred to as bladderless. Double bags are normally easier to repair if damaged, while single bags offer reduced bulk and lower drag.

In any BC, the inflator hose should be large and attached high on the collar for easy inflation and deflation. The power and oral inflator buttons should be easy to operate either with or without gloves, and easy to recognize. Pockets and hose retainers should be conveniently located to help secure and organize your equipment.

Buoyancy Compensator Use

It is recommended that you always dive with some form of buoyancy compensation device. Besides being one of the most useful diving tools, it is a valuable emergency device. By having your BC partially inflated on the surface, using energy to stay there is unnecessary because the buoyancy compensator is doing the work your fins would.

Filling a BC with a mechanical inflator is easy, but you should also learn to fill it orally in case of an inflator failure. A bobbing technique is one of the easiest and safest methods. Simply kick to clear the surface, take a deep breath, press the button on the oral inflator, and blow into the BC. You will sink slightly during blowing, but when you have finished, just kick back to clear the surface for another big breath of air and repeat the procedure. You will establish good positive buoyancy after two or three breaths. Oral inflation can be done at depth by first breathing from the regulator, then blowing into the oral inflator in much the same manner, as illustrated in Fig. 2-23.

The technique for deflating the BC varies according to its design. On compensators without dump valves, the inflator hose is held above the BC and the deflator button is depressed as shown in Fig. 2-24. This allows air to easily escape. On BCs that incorporate a dump valve, the deflation mechanism is opened, and, since the valve is usually located at the highest point on the compensator, air escapes easily, unless you are head down.

To establish neutral buoyancy under water, inflate your BC either mechanically or orally until you begin to rise. Then deflate it until you hang suspended. Using this technique together with controlling air in your lungs, enables you to maintain a state of neutral buoyancy throughout any dive at any depth. When you are ready to

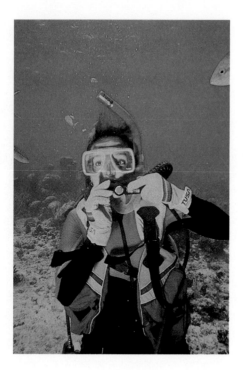

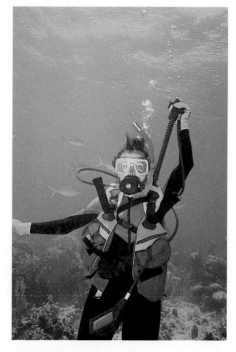

Fig. 2-23 In the event of inflator failure the BC can be orally inflated even at depth.

Fig. 2-24 Deflating the BC by using the oral inflator/deflator mechanism.

ascend, assure that you are neutrally buoyant and begin a controlled swimming ascent. As you ascend, release air from the BC to maintain a controlled rate of ascent.

Care and Maintenance of the Buoyancy Compensator

After every dive, fill the buoyancy compensator with a small amount of fresh water, inflate the BC with air, and slosh the water around, as shown in Fig. 2-25. Hold the BC upside down and open the oral inflator valve to let the water run out. Just before it is completely empty, taste the water and make sure it is clean. If it tastes salty, repeat the procedure. If the BC has a CO_2 cartridge, remove it and let the water flow through the opening of the mechanism to clean it. Again, taste the water to make certain all salt has been flushed.

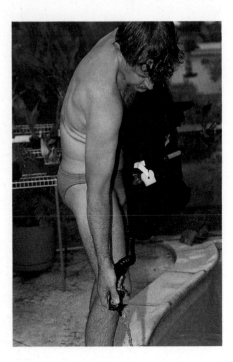

Fig. 2-25 *Following each dive, the inside of the BC should be rinsed out before the outer surface is cleaned.*

After the inside is clean, rinse the outside of the BC, taking special care to clean push-button valves, inflation mechanisms, and other parts. Lubricate the CO_2 cartridge threads and puncture disc with white all-purpose grease or some other kind of waterproof material to prevent corrosion.

Test for leaks by inflating the BC and submerging it in the bathtub, sink, or swimming pool. Look for tiny air bubbles. Repair any leaks before the next dive. When you store the BC, leave it half full of air to keep the insides from sticking together.

With proper care, your buoyancy compensator, weight belt, and wet suit will work together as a warmth-and-buoyancy control team for many years. Take care of it and it will take care of you.

3

Breathing Underwater

- Cylinder
- Regulator
- Buddy Breathing
- Buddy System

OBJECTIVES

At the conclusion of Chapter 3, you will be able to:

1. Name the two principal materials used in the manufacture of scuba tanks.
2. State how frequently your scuba tank should be visually inspected.
3. State how frequently your scuba tank should be hydrostatically tested.
4. Explain the meaning of markings required on scuba tanks.
5. Begin the regulator selection process.
6. Explain the need for and placement of an "octopus" regulator.
7. State the air source alternatives to an octopus regulator.
8. Explain and demonstrate the steps in attaching a regulator to a tank.
9. Show how to place a regulator in your mouth and clear the regulator.
10. Explain the purpose of the buddy system.

KEY TERMS

Tank	CTC	DOT
First stage	Second stage	"O" ring
Hydrotest	Ambient pressure	Diaphragm
Purge button	Dust cap	SPG
Gauge pressure	Absolute pressure	

The skin diver is constantly reminded that underwater excursions are limited by breath-holding capabilities. In what seems to be just a few moments, the skin diver making a dive must return to the surface for more air. The problem of staying underwater for longer periods of time was solved many years before skin diving became a popular sport.

Archeologists tell us that the Neanderthal, a primitive human, dove for food. As early as 4,500 B.C., diving had become an industry supplying communities with food and pearls. The Greeks, from their ancient civilization to the present day, have been commercial sponge divers.

History is replete with stories of divers being used in military applications. During the Trojan War, 1194 to 1184 B.C., divers were used to sabotage enemy ships by damaging ship hulls with drills and by cutting mooring lines.

Stories of diving with equipment were recorded long before the advent of modern diving equipment. It is said that Alexander the Great once dove in a diving bell. Leonardo da Vinci designed diving equipment that included a snorkel and fins. Early use of the diving bell was recorded in the sixteenth century. Edmund Halley, for whom the comet was named and an astronomer by profession, invented a diving bell supplied with air. (See Fig. 3-1.)

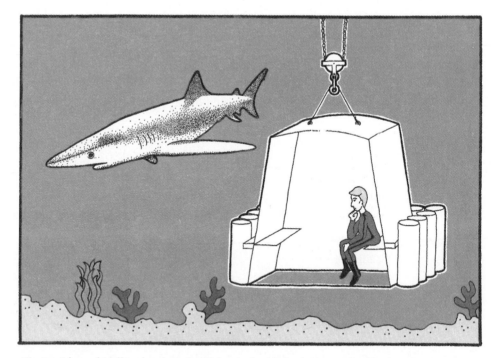

Fig. 3-1 *Edmund Halley developed a diving bell with fresh air supplied by weighted barrels of air.*

Early diving dress—which we today know as "hard hat" diving dress—was developed in the early nineteenth century. It has continued to improve to this day.

While using free diving techniques, snorkels, diving bells, and diving suits, the diver is still limited by breath-holding ability or by an attachment to a surface supply of air. Man has continually sought to be freer in the underwater environment.

An early step in the direction of this freedom came in 1865 when Frenchmen Benoit Rouquayrol and Auguste Denayrouze made public their diving apparatus, which allowed divers to store a small amount of compressed air in a tank on the back, disconnect the air supply hose from the surface, and walk freely about. (See Fig. 3-2.) Significant in the Rouquayrol-Denayrouze invention was the development of a regulator which controlled the flow of air to the diver's mouth. Similar to the "one small step" taken by the Apollo astronauts on the moon, what an exciting event that early step of underwater freedom must have been!

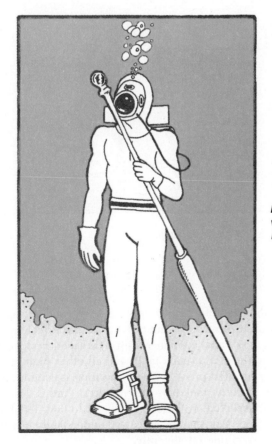

Fig. 3-2 *Predecessor of modern scuba was the 1865 aerophore invention of Rouquayrol and Denayrouze.*

The next significant step toward underwater freedom came from a French inventor, Georges Comheines, who developed a semiautomatic regulator attached to a tank of pressurized air. This apparatus was similar to the breathing apparatus used by firemen. Comheines died during one of his early dives that made use of the invention.

In 1943, Emile Gagnan and Jacques Cousteau unveiled their Aqualung, a device that supplied air from a portable tank to a diver at exactly the right pressure necessary for the diver's depth. (See Fig. 3-3.)

At last, with the advent of the Cousteau-Gagnan invention, man had the ability to carry a reasonable quantity of air and inhale that air in just the right amount regardless of depth. Modifications and improvements on this equipment have enhanced the freedom to explore and enjoy the underwater world.

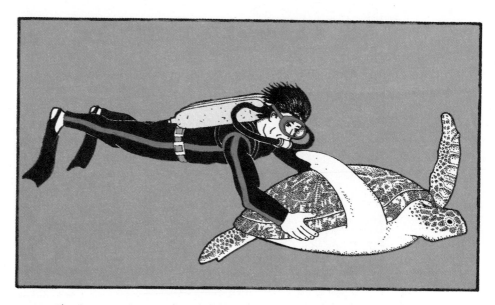

Fig. 3-3 *The Cousteau/Gagnan diving apparatus.*

SCUBA TANKS

The scuba tank (sometimes referred to as cylinders) used by sport divers has changed little since Cousteau made his first dive with the Aqualung system. It is a simple device—a seamless metal container with a threaded neck holding a valve.

The manufacture and use of a scuba tank, and all other high-pressure gas containers, is a carefully controlled process. From the time it is built to precise specifications in the factory until the tank fails the hydrotests and is destroyed, the tank is regularly tested and inspected. It would be difficult to find, let alone buy, a new scuba tank that is not good. You should, however, understand tanks well enough to select, use, and take care of one intelligently.

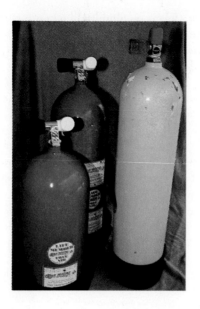

Fig. 3-4 *Various scuba tanks.*

Selecting a Tank

The first two decisions to make when selecting a tank concern size and materials. Tank sizes range from 10 cubic feet to 120 cubic feet. Smaller tanks are lighter and easier for young or lightweight divers. The tanks used most often are shown in Fig. 3-4. The 71.2 cubic-foot steel (usually called a "seventy-two") and the 80 cubic-foot aluminum are the most common size tanks used by sport divers.

The *seventy-two* is a good compromise between weight and air capacity. It weighs about 28 to 35 pounds, depending on whether it is empty or full. It is a little over 2 feet long and about 7 inches wide, and is designed to hold air at a maximum of 2,250 to 3,000 pounds per square inch gauge (psig) pressure, depending on design.

A full seventy-two contains about the same amount of air as a common telephone booth. How long will that air last? The answer depends on depth, lung capacity, activity level, water temperature, and other factors that are discussed in Chapter 8.

The aluminum 80 contains 10 percent more air than the seventy-two at normal working pressures, yet weighs about the same. Slightly larger in height and diameter, it holds 3,000 psig. Because of its buoyancy characteristics, a diver should carry at least 3 pounds more weight, to be neutrally buoyant, than would be carried with the seventy-two.

Until 1970, all sport diving tanks were made of steel. Since that time, they have also been made of aluminum alloy. The main difference between steel and aluminum is the way the two metals corrode; rust forms on steel, while aluminum oxide or aluminum hydroxide forms on aluminum.

When a metal corrodes, oxygen combines with it to form a new substance. Rust is much softer than steel, so it crumbles and flakes off.

A gray powder, aluminum oxide, forms on aluminum when it combines with oxygen. Both corrosion products tend to fall free into the tank and, if extensive, may pose a danger by blocking the valve stem. While moisture remains, aluminum oxide is usually found in its hydroxide form clinging to the tank wall.

The oxidation process happens faster when water or water vapor is present; salt in the water speeds the process even more. With oxygen, water, and salt, corrosion can eat through a steel tank wall.

Both steel and aluminum tanks can be used for many years if they are kept clean and dry, inside and out.

Warning: Aluminum tanks exposed to fire or heated to temperatures in excess of 300° F should not be filled with compressed air. The same applies to those tanks stripped of paint with catalytic paint strippers.

Do not modify or alter a tank in any way. Tanks which have been refinished by unapproved methods and/or subjected to high temperatures should be hydrostatically tested before filling to preclude rupturing during use which could, in turn, cause serious injury or loss of life.

What to Look for in a Tank

Coatings

There are a number of inside and outside coatings for scuba tanks that protect them and/or make them more attractive.

All steel tanks are galvanized to protect outside surfaces from moisture and air—two elements necessary for rust. Steel tanks are not lined with zinc inside since zinc can be toxic in heavy doses. Only the outside of the tank is galvanized.

Vinyl and epoxy coatings are sometimes painted over the zinc coating for color and additional protection, but if any of these coatings are punctured or scratched, rust may form underneath. Ordinary paint is not durable enough to either protect or beautify a steel tank for any length of time. Epoxy paint in the past was sometimes used to line the inside of steel and aluminum tanks. It protects the bare metal from corrosive effects of air and water, but the coating works only if the epoxy maintains a perfect seal over the steel. Moisture can penetrate underneath the epoxy even through a tiny hole. Since this frequently happens, rust forms under the coating where you cannot see it, and the epoxy must then be removed in order to clean the tank of rust.

Tank Markings

Like all high-pressure containers, scuba tanks must conform to regulations set by the Canadian Transport Commission (CTC) and the U.S. Department of Transportation (DOT) for the manufacturing, transporting, and testing of scuba tanks. All tanks manufactured in the United States must have "DOT" or "CTC/DOT" stamped on the shoulder, along with a series of other markings. The other markings are numbers, letters, and symbols that describe and identify the tank and also provide a record of testing validations. The meanings of these markings are shown in Fig. 3-5. Tanks made before 1982 have somewhat different markings because of the regulations existing at that time. Very old steel tanks may have "ICC" (Interstate Commerce Commission) instead of the newer "DOT." Older aluminum tanks bear a spe-

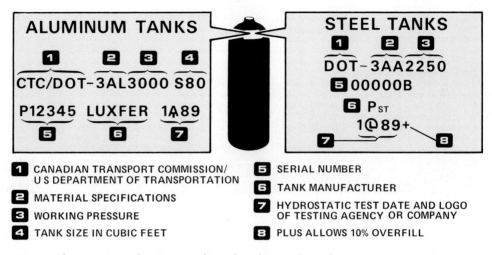

ALUMINUM TANKS		**STEEL TANKS**	

CTC/DOT-3AL3000 S80

P12345 LUXFER 1A89

DOT-3AA2250
00000B
Pst
1Q89+

1 CANADIAN TRANSPORT COMMISSION/ U S DEPARTMENT OF TRANSPORTATION

2 MATERIAL SPECIFICATIONS

3 WORKING PRESSURE

4 TANK SIZE IN CUBIC FEET

5 SERIAL NUMBER

6 TANK MANUFACTURER

7 HYDROSTATIC TEST DATE AND LOGO OF TESTING AGENCY OR COMPANY

8 PLUS ALLOWS 10% OVERFILL

Fig. 3-5 *The meanings of various markings found on scuba tanks.*

cial permit or exemption number where the 3AL mark is now placed. Tank volume appears on most models.

Without correct markings, a tank is not safe. Reputable dive stores will not fill these tanks. When buying used equipment, ensure that the tank has the appropriate markings.

Tank Valves

Tanks most commonly used in scuba are pressurized to not more than 3,000 psig, and have one of two kinds of valves at the top to turn the air on or off. The valve remains in place continuously, except for tank inspections.

The non-reserve, or "K" valve as it is usually called, is a simple on-and-off valve.

The "J," or constant reserve, has an extra lever connected to a special spring-loaded reserve mechanism which provides a warning that the tank is about to run out of air. The reserve valve allows air to flow until the pressure inside the tank falls to about 300 psig. Then the spring pressure shuts off the air flow. Pulling down the reserve lever opens the valve manually so the diver can use the remaining 300 psig of air for the ascent. Because of the additional mechanical parts and costs involved in the "J" valve along with current standards that all divers should be diving with a submersible pressure gauge, the "J" valve is seen less frequently but may still be encountered. The two types of tank valves are shown in Figs. 3-6 and 3-7.

The small "O" ring that surrounds the air outlet on the tank valve forms the seal between the tank valve and the regulator yoke. Without the "O" ring, a seal cannot be made, so always carry an extra one. (If the design of your regulator allows it, you may be able to carry an extra "O" ring between the yolk screw and the yolk on your regulator.) "O" rings vary in size so be sure your spare is compatible with the tank you are using.

With the development of stronger steel alloys and the modification of basic tank design, newer tanks that can be filled to pressures greater than 3,000 psig have come into the sport scuba market. However, these higher pressures exceed the de-

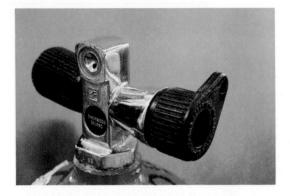

Fig. 3-6 *The "J" tank valve.*

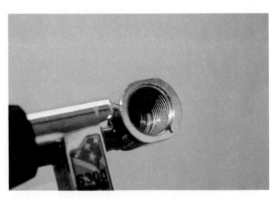

Fig. 3-7 *The "K" tank valve.*

sign limits of standard tank valves and regulator connections. Several tank/regulator combinations in the marketplace utilize a DIN connection and have multiple "O" rings for more secure connections at pressures over 3,000 psig. This DIN connection system is illustrated in Fig. 3-8.

A frangible burst disc assembly in a valve is a safety feature to prevent the tank from being excessively overpressurized. The burst disc is designed to give way at some point between 125 and 166 percent of the tank's working pressure to let the air escape harmlessly and avoid tank rupture. Valves without a frangible disc are illegal; without this safety feature, a filled tank overheated by fire, the sun, or some other source could explode.

Valves are made of relatively soft naval brass and may be damaged by careless attempts at their removal, a task better left to trained technicians. A defective valve may cause you to believe the tank is empty when air pressure remains. Because of this, some valves have a small safety hole drilled into the threads which lets any pressurized tank air escape before you have unscrewed the valve more than a few turns. Most tank valves do not have this protection.

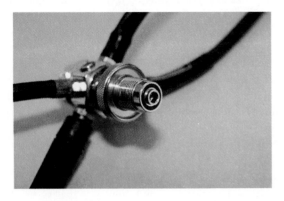

Fig. 3-8 *The DIN high-pressure cylinder valve for high-pressure systems.*

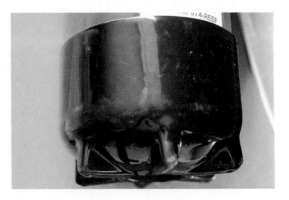

Fig. 3-9 *Tank boots protect tank, pool deck, boat deck, and floor.*

The valve pigtail extends into the tank and helps keep water, corrosion product, or other contaminants that should not be in your tank out of your regulator. Small amounts of water or contaminants are trapped in the tank by a 2-inch valve pigtail. Larger amounts of contaminants may enter into the valve air passageways and damage all equipment through which the foul air passes.

Tank Boots

Tank boots, like those shown in Fig. 3-9, are designed to protect the tank, pool, floor, and boat deck from collision damage. A boot allows steel tanks to stand upright, but, since most tanks are easily knocked over, they should not be left standing unattended when they might fall and cause damage or injury. This is especially true on a boat or in a high-traffic area.

All installed boots, whether of open or closed design, trap some water against the tank. Retained salt water may lead to serious corrosion of the tank where trapped. Because of this, boots must be removed regularly to clean and inspect the tank surface for evidence of significant corrosion damage. Nongalvanized steel tanks are especially vulnerable to this corrosion. Tank boots should be self-draining insofar as possible.

Backpack

The purpose of the backpack or the backpack component of the buoyancy compensator is to securely attach the scuba tank to your back. It is unusual today to find backpacks utilized separately, as they are usually an integral part of the buoyancy compensator.

When you select a backpack, make sure everything on the pack is made of non-corroding materials. The backpack is normally equipped with a quick-release fastening at the waist for easy jettisoning of the tank during rescue. The tank retaining band holds the tank to the backpack. The retaining bands can have either adjustable buckles or Velcro straps. Adjustable tank bands are designed to fit several tank sizes. (See Fig. 3-10.)

Make sure the tank band is tight before each dive. Bands made of nylon webbing tend to loosen when the band gets wet. If possible wet the tank band prior to putting the BC on the tank. Adjust the backpack so that your head does not hit the tank valve when you lean back. After securing the backpack, lay the tank on its side

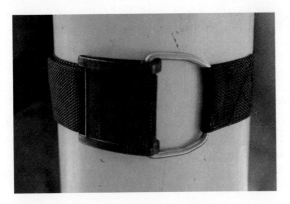

Fig. 3-10 Adjustable tank straps.

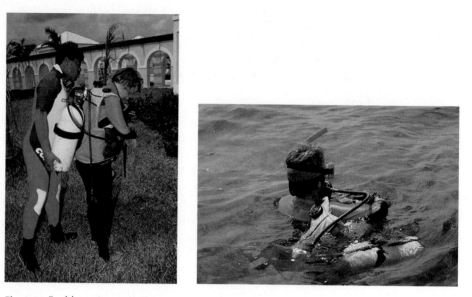

Fig. 3-11 *Buddy assist to putting on scuba.*

Fig. 3-12 *Putting on scuba on surface.*

until you are ready to put it on, or secure it in the tank racks found on most dive boats. Tanks left free-standing can fall over and cause damage to a boat or pool deck or injury to nearby people.

There are many different ways to don (put on) a scuba tank. Your buddy can hold it for you while you slip your arms through the shoulder straps, fasten the shoulder and waist buckles, and adjust the straps. (See Fig. 3-11.) A variation on this technique is to stand the tank on a table, gunwale of a boat, or other platform instead of having your buddy hold it up. Then hold it with one hand while you slip the other arm through the shoulder straps and continue, as you would with a buddy.

Another method for donning jacket and low-profile scuba units is shown in Fig. 3-12. While resting at the surface, position the tank and slightly inflated BC assembly with the front facing you. Leave shoulder straps buckled but loose, and put your regulator in your mouth, if you wish. Then, slip your right arm through the shoulder strap and slip the assembly on as you would a jacket. Make sure the hoses and straps are not tangled before you secure the waist strap or cummerbund, and tighten the shoulder straps. Your instructor may show you other methods appropriate to your own equipment style.

Care and Maintenance of the Tank

Scuba tank care, for the most part, means keeping moisture out of the tank. As with all diving equipment, the exterior should be rinsed thoroughly with fresh water after each dive and washed with mild soap and water when it gets dirty. To help keep water out of the tank, keep no less than 100 psig in the tank at all times, except when travelling by plane (see below).

When carrying a tank in a car, lash it down, block it, or secure it in a scuba tank transport device and either lay it sideways on the floor or lengthwise in the trunk, with the valve toward the rear. Wrap the valve in a thick cloth, such as a beach towel, to protect the valve and the car.

When preparing to transport a tank by airplane, slowly discharge the air (take 30 minutes or more) and leave the valve open. Some airlines even require the tank valve to be removed.

Tanks scheduled for long-term storage should be visually inspected to ensure there is no water, corrosion, or other contamination inside. A tank is best secured standing in a cool, dry location. Steel tanks should be stored with low pressure, while aluminum tanks are stored either filled or emptied with the valve open to avoid explosion of a partially filled tank exposed to fire. A full tank exposed to fire will safely discharge its air through the frangible burst disc. Both types of tanks may be filled for short-term storage.

Visual Inspections (Internal and External)

A thorough visual inspection at least once each year by a professional inspector is the best way to make sure that a tank is clean, corrosion-free, and safe between hydrostatic tests. A visual inspection is called for whenever the tank shows obvious physical damage or the air coming from the tank has an odor. Besides inspecting both steel and aluminum tanks for damage caused by general pitting or line corrosion, inspectors will also look for contaminates such as carbon, oil, or water injected by air compressors and charging stations.

Certain aluminum tanks made before 1990 must also undergo a yearly special visual examination for a possible cracking defect in their shoulder and threads. A flawed tank may be returned to the manufacturer for replacement.

Most scuba shops will not fill a tank without evidence that it has been visually inspected within the past year.

In caring for a tank, remember that it is easier to prevent contamination than to clean it out. The prime prevention is to never let all the tank air out of the tank. If it is emptied underwater, its valve should be shut immediately to keep water from entering. It should also be shut when a regulator is attached and the purge valve is open, because that, too, is a direct open route to the tank for the entry of contamination.

Water can also appear inside the tank if air is released too quickly. For example, suppose you want to store a full tank for several months. If you open the valve far enough, most of the air will escape in a matter of minutes. Upon escape from the tank, the air expands and, since gasses cool when they expand (refrigerators and air conditioners are based on this principle), the tank itself will become very cool. If water vapor is present in any quantity in the tank, the vapor will condense on the inside of the tank. This water vapor might be present in air if the air was not properly dried during filling. To prevent possible water condensation, slowly let all the air out of the tank when you are emptying or nearly emptying a tank for any reason.

Another way of putting water in the tank is to connect a tank filler to a tank with a wet valve and blow it in with the air.

Between annual visual inspections, routinely look, smell, and listen to your tank for hints of water inside.

1. **Look.** Turn the valve on and check the air coming out. Damp air is white. Dry air is clear and invisible.
2. **Smell.** Pure, clean air does not smell. If the air from your tank smells damp and metallic, there could be water, oil, or corrosion inside.
3. **Listen.** Put your ear next to the tank. Turn the tank upside down so that anything inside will fall to the other end. A clean, dry tank does not make a sound.

If you have cause to suspect your tank has water in it, have it visually inspected immediately. Otherwise, have it inspected once a year. A full-service dive store is equipped to inspect and test tanks and is usually in contact with a hydrotesting firm that services all kinds of high pressure cylinders. Tanks that have been visually inspected bear stickers similar to what is shown in Fig. 3-13.

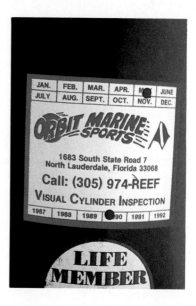

Fig. 3-13 Tanks bear stickers similar to the above after passing visual inspection.

Visual inspection begins when the inspector examines the tank's exterior after removing all outside accoutrements. The inspector will look for any dents, bulges, or corrosion, then let all air slowly escape from the tank and remove the tank valve to inspect inside. A special light or series of lights is required to conduct a proper internal inspection for corrosion, water, salt, flaked epoxy linings, and especially pits or rough and scaly surfaces. These must be cleaned out for continued use of the tank.

To clean the tank, the inspector fills a steel tank half full with some type of abrasive material, such as carbide or aluminum oxide chips. After capping, the tank is laid down on two rotating rollers to tumble and make the abrasive chips scrape the inside of the tank clean so the extent of actual damage can be seen clearly. Some hydrotesting firms use a rotating chain or sandblasting machine instead of chips to clean the inside, but these methods are neither thorough nor complete. Likewise, harsh chemicals should never be put inside a tank because lingering fumes can be toxic.

After tumbling, the inspector examines the inside again to see if corrosion was only on the surface or was more serious. Tank damage will be compared to maximum allowable guidelines. If exceeded, the tank must be condemned and removed from service.

Hydrostatic Testing

At least every 5 years a tank must be hydrostatically tested for metal integrity by a federally licensed facility, which will stamp a federal designation number on the tank as evidence of a successful test. This test of metal integrity assesses certain conditions beyond the scope of an annual visual inspection. Most dive stores can contract for this service.

After a complete visual inspection, the hydrotest begins. It is designed to measure the elasticity of the metal within the tank. The tank is filled with water, connected to a high-pressure water pump, and submerged in a sealed container that is also filled with water. Water is forced into the tank at five-thirds (three-halves for certain tanks) of its working pressure, which makes the tank expand.

The testing pressure is held for 30 seconds, then released to let the expanded tank return to normal. To pass the test, the permanent expansion cannot be more than 10 percent of total expansion.

What happens if the tank ruptures during the hydrostatic test? Nothing much. Unlike a tank filled with air, a water-filled tank is not explosive. If the tank should break, it relieves the water pressure almost immediately without much expansion.

After the hydrotest, the tank must be thoroughly dried with warm air from the inside. Usually, warm air is blown into the tank through a tube. Heating the tank from the outside does not work—it causes steam to form which later condenses in the tank when it cools.

Hydrotesting is safe, reliable, and cheap, especially when you consider the insurance it provides. It is comforting to know your tank will hold almost twice the amount of internal pressure you will ever put into it. Feel free to hydrotest your tank more often than the once every 5 years required in the United States.

Although rarely done, a more complex evaluation—the elastic expansion test— may be performed on steel tanks; it is typically done at the same time a tank is hydrostatically tested. Those tanks which pass may be overfilled by 10 percent for the coming 5-year period. The allowable overpressure is noted by a plus ("+") mark following the hydrotest mark.

THE REGULATOR

Squeezing air into a tank at over 200 times atmospheric pressure is easy, compared to taking the same quantity of air out and delivering it to a diver at a usable pressure while submerged.

That is why the demand regulator was so important to the growth of diving. With a scuba regulator, the diver receives just the right amount of air, at the right pressure, and at the right time.

Selecting a Regulator

Regulators are finely adjusted, precise pieces of equipment designed for reliability and durability. Just like automobiles, regulators vary in how well they perform. All regulators have some measure of breathing resistance but better ones offer less resistance than others.

Breathing resistance is caused by a number of things. Hard work and cold water make you breathe much harder. Most regulators have very little breathing resistance at the surface. The real test occurs near the end of a long hard dive, in deep water. Here, heavy breathing and increased water pressure, under conditions of low tank pressure, tend to increase breathing resistance.

What makes one regulator easier to breathe through than another? Having a basic understanding of regulator operation will help you understand the reasons for differences.

Modern regulators reduce the tank pressure to breathable pressures in two stages. The first stage reduces the high tank pressure to about 140 psi over ambient pressure (pressure of the "surrounding" environment). The second stage further reduces that pressure to a workable breathing pressure of essentially ambient pressure. This two-stage system has proven effective, smooth, and reliable for over 30 years.

The single-hose, two-stage regulator, shown in Fig. 3-14, is almost the only type used in sport diving. It provides an automatically regulated delivery of air with the mouthpiece on the second stage.

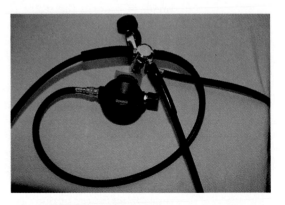

Fig. 3-14 *The single-hose, two-stage regulator is the standard in sport scuba diving.*

The first stage of the single-hose, two-stage regulator comes in two basic designs: diaphragm and piston. Excellent regulators are available in either design. Modern regulator first stages are "balanced" so that low tank pressure has a reduced influence on how the regulator breathes; yet low tank pressures at depth will still have an effect on breathing effort. Other regulators are labelled unbalanced and the work involved in breathing as tank pressure drops gets significantly greater than with balanced regulators.

In a balanced first stage, tank pressure is not allowed to contact any surface area that affects first-stage valve movement. The valve moves only in response to inha-

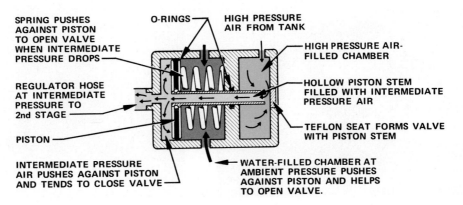

SPRING PUSHES AGAINST PISTON TO OPEN VALVE WHEN INTERMEDIATE PRESSURE DROPS

O-RINGS

HIGH PRESSURE AIR FROM TANK

HIGH PRESSURE AIR-FILLED CHAMBER

REGULATOR HOSE AT INTERMEDIATE PRESSURE TO 2nd STAGE

HOLLOW PISTON STEM FILLED WITH INTERMEDIATE PRESSURE AIR

PISTON

TEFLON SEAT FORMS VALVE WITH PISTON STEM

INTERMEDIATE PRESSURE AIR PUSHES AGAINST PISTON AND TENDS TO CLOSE VALVE

WATER-FILLED CHAMBER AT AMBIENT PRESSURE PUSHES AGAINST PISTON AND HELPS TO OPEN VALVE.

Fig. 3-15 *A cross-section of the balanced piston first stage.*

lation effort of the diver as influenced by a reduction in intermediate pressure. In an unbalanced first stage, the tank pressure helps open the first-stage valve. When tank pressure falls, it provides less help, which results in harder inhalation. A spring in the first stage sets the intermediate pressure. (See Fig. 3-15.)

Both balanced and unbalanced first stages deliver air to the second stage at a relatively constant pressure, controlled by a spring in the first stage. Because of this, the second stage can be tuned to the constant pressure provided by the first stage. Since the size of the orifice through which breathing air passes is constant, breathing resistance will increase with depth, due to an increase in air density.

The pressure to the second stage stays at a constant value, usually about 140 psi over ambient pressure. This intermediate pressure is further reduced to ambient by the second stage.

Many second-stage regulators are "downstream" lever-action valve regulators. Downstream means that the second-stage air valve opens with the intermediate pressure, which tends to push the valve open. If the valve fails to close, it will "free flow" or leak air through the mouthpiece. You can still breathe from a free-flowing regulator but the leaking air reduces your air supply.

Most single-hose demand regulators have a rubber diaphragm in the second stage, which helps a diver open the second-stage air valve with little effort. (See Figs. 3-16 and 3-17.)

Some second stages manufactured today can even be "tuned" during a dive to match your personal breathing needs.

A high-quality regulator is important. Regardless of design features, your regulator is your lifeline; it supplies the air you breathe. Any regulator gives you air to sustain life, but there are differences between high-quality and low-quality models.

The differences include breathing ease, durability, and dependability. Actually breathing from the regulator in the water is the best way to evaluate its breathing ease. The availability of parts and service, plus the "real world" track record of any regulator model, helps indicate durability and dependability. Consider these factors before you select a regulator.

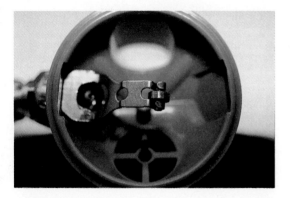

Fig. 3-16 *This close-up shows the valve lever that controls entry of intermediate pressure into the second stage with the tip of the lever always in contact with the undersurface of the diaphragm.*

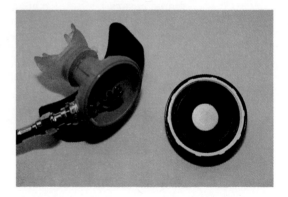

Fig. 3-17 *Close-up of the diaphragm. This is the critical area relative to breathing forces required to open and close the downstream valve.*

Reserve Options

Octopus Regulator

Beginning in the 1960s, resort instructors and cave divers started attaching an extra second stage to an extra low-pressure port on the regulator's first stage. This octopus regulator is shown in Fig. 3-18.

The octopus regulator was attached for two reasons. The first is that it provides an independent mouthpiece for emergency buddy breathing. The second, and less important, is that it provides a backup system in case the primary second stage fails.

During a dive, the octopus regulator is best kept secured yet readily available: secured, so that it does not drag on the bottom or get snagged by obstructions; and available so it can be put into use without hassle. Though some instructors advocate leaving it loose, others advocate attaching it in a "golden triangle" placement of essential equipment on your chest, including the octopus or other alternate air

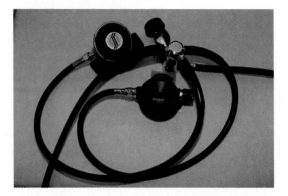

Fig. 3-18 *Regulator system with octopus second stage attached.*

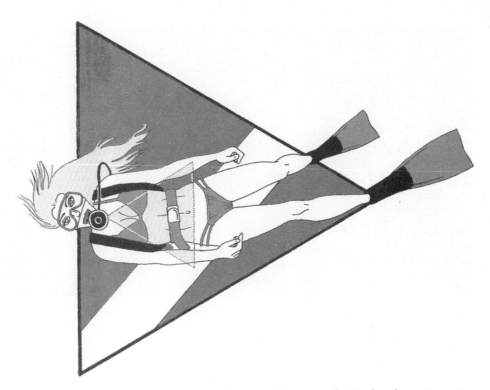

Fig. 3-19 *The "golden triangle" concept relative to placement of critical scuba equipment.*

source. (See Fig. 3-19.) A BC inflator system that incorporates an octopus follows the golden triangle concept as can a pop-release connection for your octopus.

The alternate air source, like the buoyancy compensator and submersible pressure gauge, has become a standard piece of equipment for most scuba divers.

Separate Alternate Air Sources

Some divers advocate carrying an entirely separate first and second stage along with its own air supply as an alternative to the octopus. Figs. 3-20 and 3-21 show several types of completely independent emergency sources of air that can supply a diver with enough air to return immediately to the surface in the event of primary regulator failure, or might even be used in a buddy emergency. Though principally designed as self-rescue devices, the advantage of these devices is that they can actually be given to a distressed diver without having to remain in close contact, which is hazardous in times of panic.

First-Stage Reserves

With proper dive planning, a diver can easily finish every dive and have air left to cope with unforeseen problems at the surface. Though not readily apparent today, early systems warning the diver of low air supply included the "R" (restricted ori-

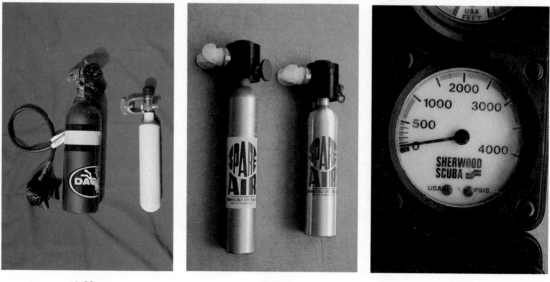

3-20   3-21   3-22

Fig. 3-20 *Two forms of secondary tank, each of which will be used with its own first-stage and second-stage regulators.*

Fig. 3-21 *A popular alternate air source for use in emergencies, which is primarily a self-rescue tool but may be given to a buddy in an emergency.*

Fig. 3-22 *The submersible pressure gauge, your "fuel gauge" for breathing air.*

fice) tank valve, the "J" tank valve, and audible alarms on either the first-stage regulator or in the tank valve.

The "R" valve restricted air flow at various low pressures to warn the diver of low air by creating greater breathing resistance at trigger levels.

The "J" valve warns the diver when the air supply drops to between 300 and 600 psi. To provide these warnings, the valve has to be set before the dive. The "J" valve has a lever which has to be in the up ("start dive") position until pulled down to use the reserve air. If it is accidentally knocked down ("on reserve") or if the diver does not set it up before the dive, it does not give a warning.

The audible, or sonic, reserve built into the first stage of some regulators or tank valves buzzed or clicked with each inhalation when the air supply was low. These required no predive setup, nor could it be unset during a dive.

Both the reserve valve and the audible alarm systems warned a diver but they did not give any other pressure information about air supply. The submersible pressure gauge (SPG) (Fig. 3-22) does and has essentially replaced the reserve valve or the audible alarm, since it tells you approximately how much air you have left in your tank at any time. It is standard equipment for all scuba divers.

The SPG is like a fuel gauge in a car—it tells you nothing unless you look at it—so you should check your tank pressure gauge regularly during a dive and always be aware of air remaining. A safe diver never dives without one.

The SPG is connected to a high pressure port in your regulator first stage so it will be able to monitor tank pressure directly. It should be attached by a dive store professional, unless you are fully trained in dive equipment assembly and disassembly. The SPG when attached helps you constantly monitor your air supply and make informed decisions about your dive plan underwater.

Using the Regulator

A regulator is quite rugged because the first stage is made of metal, and the second-stage regulator is made of either metal or high-strength plastic. The inside with its precise clearances is best kept as clean as possible; you should protect the mouthpiece and exhaust valve from sand and dirt, and always keep a dust cap firmly in the first-stage regulator yoke when not in use, as shown in Fig. 3-23. Tank valves and regulators with DIN connections are covered for protection as shown in Fig. 3-24. Do not store a regulator attached to the tank valve because that flattens the tank valve "O" ring and exposes the regulator to damage from falling. Remove it as soon as you finish diving.

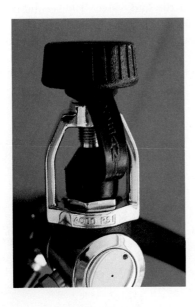

Fig. 3-23 It is important to put the dust cap in place on the first stage regulator yoke when the regulator is not in use.

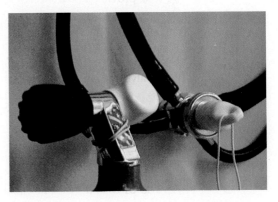

Fig. 3-24 Dust protection on high-pressure DIN connections.

Assembly

Attaching a regulator first stage to the tank is a basic skill for scuba divers. Check that the air opening in the tank valve is clear and dry even though it has been stored after refilling with either a tank-valve cover or tape over the opening. Follow the steps illustrated in Figs. 3-25 through 3-31 when you attach a yoke-equipped regulator to your tank. (*Note:* Steps 1 through 5 differ for a DIN regulator in that screwing the first stage into the tank valve replaces the actions involving the yoke.)

1. Begin with the tank in front of you and the backpack on the opposite side and attached to the tank. This should place the tank valve opening away from you and the tank valve knob on your right side. Hold the tank between your knees to steady it.

2. Momentarily open then close the tank valve to blow out any dust or moisture which may have accumulated. Make sure when you do this that you and anyone else are clear of the path of the burst of air that may escape. (See Fig. 3-25.)

3. Looking over the top of the tank valve, examine the "O" ring in the opening as shown in Fig. 3-26. If it is cracked or damaged, replace it.

4. As shown in Fig. 3-27, remove the dust cover from the first stage, then hold the second-stage regulator in your right hand and the first stage in your left hand, and put the yoke over the tank valve. The second-stage air hose is directed over your right shoulder for U.S.-made regulators.

5. In Fig. 3-28, tighten the regulator yoke screw with only two fingers until it is tight. If you tighten it too much, it will damage the "O" ring and may be difficult to remove. Check the exhaust valve of both the primary and the oc-

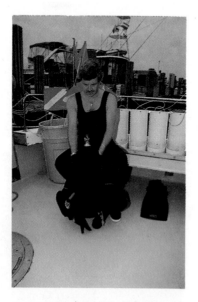

Fig. 3-25 Tank on BC with valve clear.

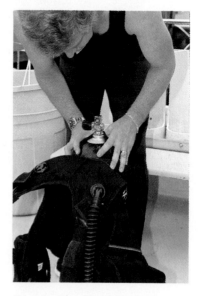

Fig. 3-26 Checking "O" ring.

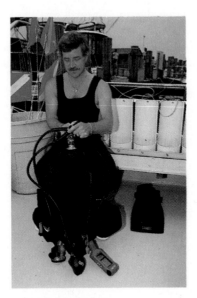

Fig. 3-27 *Place yolk over tank valve.*

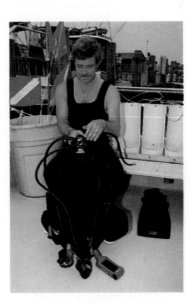

Fig. 3-28 *Tightening yolk screw.*

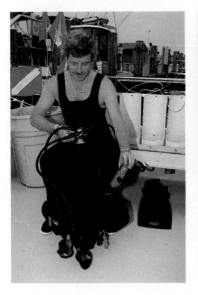

Fig. 3-29 *Turning on air—SPG faces away.*

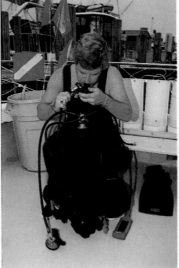

Fig. 3-30 *Checking regulators.*

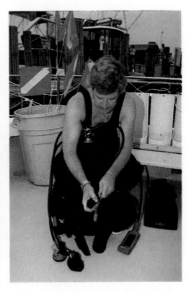

Fig. 3-31 *Connect inflator hose.*

topus second stages by trying to inhale through the regulator with the air off. If you cannot inhale, the valves are not leaking.

6. Hold the SPG face away from you as shown in Fig. 3-29, and turn the valve knob counterclockwise to turn on the air. You will feel the hose stiffen as air fills it. Gently open the valve all the way, then turn it back slightly restricting the air flow. Read the pressure to verify that the tank is filled with air. Listen for leaks. If you hear one, turn the valve off and locate the source of the leak.

7. As shown in Fig. 3-30, place the mouthpiece in your mouth, exhale first, then inhale through the primary and the octopus to make sure you can inhale and exhale through both. If you cannot exhale, the exhaust is stuck shut. Free it by blowing hard into the mouthpiece or purging the regulator with the mouthpiece blocked off.

8. Fig. 3-31, shows the diver connecting the low-pressure inflator hose to the BC.

Disassembly, Care, and Maintenance

Before disassembly, rinse the regulator thoroughly in fresh water, if possible. To remove the regulator, turn off the air and release the intermediate air pressure by purging both second stages. Remove the first stage and dry the inside of the dust cap and put it in place.

If the regulator was not already rinsed, rinse it with fresh, clean water with the dust cap in place and the purge valve not depressed before storage.

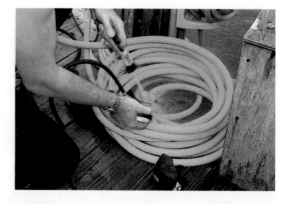

Fig. 3-32 *Rinsing the second stage after completing the dive.*

Rinsing the regulator consists of flushing water into the mouthpiece and through the exhaust ports as shown in Fig. 3-32. Be careful not to press the purge button while rinsing the second stage inside; otherwise, water may enter the air hose and contaminate it.

Store the regulator in a protective bag to prevent dust and abuse from shortening the regulator's life. Do not hang it by the regulator yoke because this will bend the hoses and weaken them where they attach to the first stage.

Regulator Clearing

If your regulator is out of your mouth underwater, for your safety you should exhale gently at all times. When out of your mouth, the mouthpiece chamber will tend to fill with water. There are two ways to clear it of water so you can inhale again: after replacing it in your mouth, either "blow" it clear or "purge" it clear.

Blasting the regulator clear is simply exhaling forcefully into it with the exhaust valve in a down position. Unlike blasting a snorkel clear, only a small puff of air is needed to completely clear a regulator. If you feel you do not have enough air in your lungs to exhale, try coughing a couple of times to clear it.

Purging, on the other hand, uses tank air to clear the regulator. With the regulator in your mouth and your tongue blocking the mouthpiece, just press the purge button momentarily as shown in Fig. 3-33. That opens the downstream valve and allows intermediate pressure air to force water out through the second-stage exhaust valve. If the tongue is not used to occlude the mouthpiece, a slight back pressure must be maintained. Failure to do either while purging the second stage may result in water from the second stage being blown into the mouth. Again, only a small amount of air is needed to completely clear the regulator.

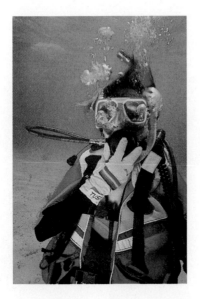

Fig. 3-33 *Clearing the second stage by use of the purge button.*

After clearing the regulator, always inhale cautiously in case there is water remaining in the mouthpiece. If there is, a gentle inhalation will allow you to get air without inhaling the water. You can then clear the regulator again to expel the remaining water.

When using a regulator underwater, breathe deeply and regularly. Do not breathe at a faster rate than normal and do not breathe more slowly to save air. As you increase your comfort, a long slow inhalation followed by a long slow exhalation will enable you to minimize breathing effort and maintain comfortable breathing.

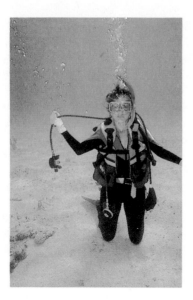

Fig. 3-34 *The diver recovers the second-stage regulator by reaching over the right shoulder and sliding the hand down the hose contacted.*

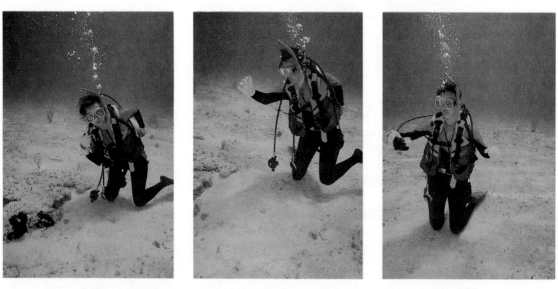

3-35   3-36   3-37

Fig. 3-35 *The diver in the vertical position leans forward and lifts the bottom of the tank, tilting it toward the right shoulder.*

Fig. 3-36 *The regulator hoses are swept up by the right arm.*

Fig. 3-37 *The regulator is recovered when the diver comes to the end of the regulator hose.*

Regulator Recovery

How do you find a lost second stage? One sure way is to reach back with your right hand to where the regulator is attached to the tank, as shown in Fig. 3-34. This may be made a little easier if you lift the bottom of your tank with your left hand and tilt the tank valve toward your right shoulder. When you find the attachment point, move your hand down the hose until it runs into the mouthpiece. Since you may grab the octopus in this process, it really does not matter which regulator supplies you with air. If you discover you have recovered your octopus, simply repeat the process and recover your primary second-stage regulator.

Another method of regulator recovery is to dip your right shoulder down, reach back behind your hip, and sweep with your right arm to catch the hose for your second stage. If in a kneeling position, you will also need to lean forward to use this recovery technique. This technique is illustrated in Figs. 3-35 through 3-37.

Either technique works in or out of the water. Normally, if the mouthpiece is not in your mouth, it will be draped over your right shoulder or hanging along the right side of the tank. If your octopus is available in its secured position, as suggested earlier, it too will be available should you lose your primary second stage.

If the normal placement of your second stage places the regulator hose under the right arm with a swivel attachment between the intermediate pressure hose and the second stage, recovering the regulator by reaching over the right shoulder with this regulator placement may be difficult; however, leaning to the right and sweeping with the right arm should do it easily.

BUDDY BREATHING

With good equipment care and dive planning, there is little chance you will ever lose your air supply. If you do, however, buddy breathing is one method of sharing your buddy's air to the surface. Another method, octopus breathing, has already been mentioned and is preferred because it is easier and safer. Two additional techniques—emergency swimming ascents and emergency buoyant ascents—are discussed in Chapter 8.

Buddy breathing is a process in which two divers share one second-stage regulator for breathing.

Buddy breathing begins when the diver who needs air—the needer—signals the diver who has air—the giver or donor—that he or she needs air.

Since the needer may be distressed or somewhat out of control because of loss of air, the donor should take control and initiate buddy breathing by offering the primary second stage to the needer. The needer takes two or three quick, large breaths from the regulator and passes it back to the donor.

The two divers then establish a deliberate breathing rhythm with each diver taking one or two breaths before passing the regulator back to the other, as shown in Figs. 3-38 through 3-40.

The donor is somewhat in front of the needer to maintain eye contact, but also off to the left to enable easy exchange of the regulator mouthpiece. The donor maintains a firm hold on the regulator at all times with the right hand but does so in such a way as to allow the needer access to the purge button. The needer holds the

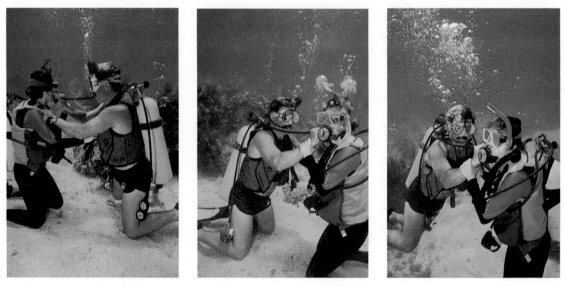

3-38   3-39   3-40

Fig. 3-38 *Divers buddy breathing. Note contact between donor and needer.*

Fig. 3-39 *Buddy breathing, opposite view. Note donor controlling regulator with needer holding donor's arm.*

Fig. 3-40 *Buddy breathing while ascending. Notice that donor keeps a constant eye on the needer and is controlling the ascent.*

donor's equipment straps with the free right hand. The donor's left hand is free to vent BCs and control ascent rate.

When linking up for air sharing, it is important to maintain contact so the buddy pair does not sink if they are in deeper open water.

Once the divers establish a breathing rhythm and have control of their position and movements, they ascend by kicking slowly and exhaling faithfully between inhalations. The ascent can be made easier if slightly positive buoyancy is maintained during the ascent. The ascent should be controlled at a leisurely rate, not rushed.

Since buddy breathing requires significant coordination between buddies, it is easy to lose track of your ascent rate, and it may be tempting to hold your breath when the regulator is not in your mouth. *When buddy breathing, make sure both you and your buddy exhale continuously when not inhaling.*

If either of you is not exhaling, stop your ascent until exhalation is resumed. Buddy breathing is a complex skill which can be developed and maintained by repeated practice for smooth use in an emergency.

Once initiated, sharing air with an octopus regulator is much easier than buddy breathing as shown in Figs. 3-41 and 3-42. Linking up, finding the octopus, and initiating air sharing are all that is involved in octopus breathing. Once the needer has the octopus mouthpiece in place, the two divers can ascend simply without any further manipulations of the regulator.

In air sharing, the diver having air may not have much left, either. You should

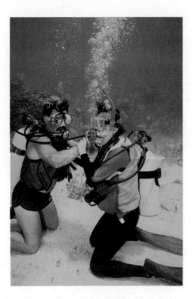

Fig. 3-41 Octopus air sharing.

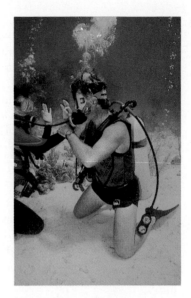

Fig. 3-42 During octopus air sharing, the divers give mutual OK signs to indicate they are comfortable and controlled enough for the ascent.

be prepared to stop air sharing at any time during an ascent and switch to an emergency swimming or buoyant ascent. Besides monitoring your buddy and the ascent rate, monitor the air supply too, so that running out of air will not be a surprise, should it happen. Although less complex than buddy breathing, octopus air sharing should be practiced routinely with new diving companions. (See Fig. 3-43.)

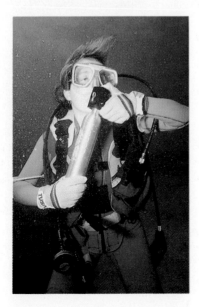

Fig. 3-43 This is how one form of alternate air source is utilized by a distressed diver or a diving companion whose primary air source is depleted.

BUDDY SYSTEM

Buddy breathing is only one small part of a broader philosophy that should be practiced on every dive you make—the buddy system. In fact, with the buddy system as an essential part of everyone's diving skills, the need for buddy breathing would essentially be eliminated. Both you and your buddy will have agreed on depth, time, and minimum air limits before the dive to ensure that you will have air left in your tanks on the surface *after* the dive.

Other aspects essential to the effective operation of the buddy system are as follows:

1. Know your buddy's gear well enough to be able to find and operate it at a moment's notice. That is especially true for the weight belt and BC releases and BC inflators for rescue or assistance purposes. (See Fig. 3-44.)
2. Know what you want to accomplish during your dive. You and your buddy should prepare and agree on the dive plan. As shown in Fig. 3-45, your buddy team should review the dive plan just before entering the water, to coordinate how you will use equipment and stay together to carry out the common goal.
3. Agree on how you will stay together, what signals to use, and what to do in case of an emergency. Try to avoid the "leader and follower" configuration since swimming shoulder-to-shoulder is easier to control. (See Fig. 3-46.) The emergencies to consider include running out of air and situations involv-

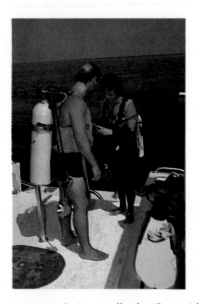

Fig. 3-44 *Being totally familiar with the placement of your buddy's equipment is very important as part of your predive activity.*

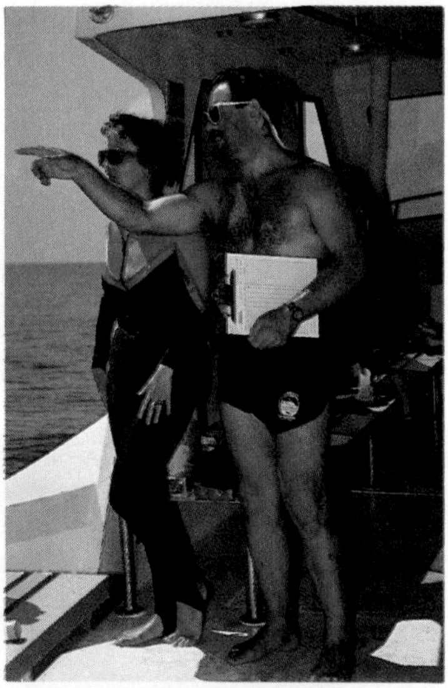

Fig. 3-45 *The diving buddies review their dive plan immediately before initiating the dive.*

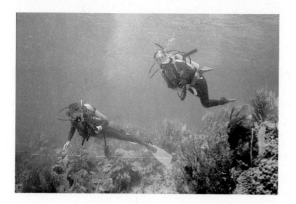

Fig. 3-46 *It is important to stay within a short distance of your buddy throughout the dive.*

ing a lost buddy, entanglement underwater, and down current from your boat or exit point.

4. Know your diving environment including entry and exit points, currents, bottom configuration, and the weather. (See also Chapters 11 and 12.)

Once in the water, you should stick with your dive plan until you are out of the water. Maintain contact with your buddy within arm's reach so you will be able to share your dive enjoyment and render aid immediately if it is needed. (First aid techniques are discussed in Chapter 7.)

SUMMARY

The self-contained breathing apparatus was little more than science fiction for over 200 years, yet almost overnight, in the middle of this century, that fiction became scientific fact. That fact, coupled with an in-depth understanding of the scuba "breathing machine" and how to use it, along with the buddy system, gives you comfortable, free access to the beautiful and exciting underwater realm.

Maintain and operate your equipment with care. Use the buddy system effectively. Plan your dives with common sense and enjoy your underwater adventures to enrich your life.

4 *Underwater Information*

- Submersible Pressure Gauge
- Underwater Timing Devices
- Depth Gauge
- Dive Computers
- Compass
- Natural Navigation

OBJECTIVES

At the conclusion of Chapter 4, you will be able to:

1. Name three beneficial features of an SPG.
2. Name three types of underwater timing devices.
3. Name four types of depth gauge.
4. Convert meters to feet and feet to meters if given different simple depth conversion problems.
5. Explain the advantage of the maximum depth indicator needle.
6. Explain the use of and place for diving computers.
7. Name three types of compasses.
8. Give the reciprocal for a compass course taken on the outbound leg of a dive.
9. Give the directions north, east, south, and west in degrees.
10. Name at least three natural navigational aids that might be used in diving.

KEY TERMS

Bezel	FSW	Outbound
Capillary	MSW	Lubber's line
Maximum depth indicator	Computer	Reciprocal

Pressure, Time, and Direction Devices

Living on land is a relatively flat, two-dimensional experience with gravity holding things in place. The position of the sun, countless clocks, convenient roads, and other landmarks help determine time and direction. Terrestrial air supply is normally unlimited.

The underwater realm, however, is relatively uncharted, three-dimensional space with gravitational restraints replaced by new options of sinking, rising, or hovering. The regular time indicators disappear. Sometimes, directions can become indistinguishable. A diver's air supply is definitely limited.

Just as a spaceman in outer space needs sophisticated instrumentation for information about the alien worlds there, so does the diver need it in the innerspace of the underwater world where survival is not possible for more than a few minutes without special life-support equipment.

SUBMERSIBLE PRESSURE GAUGE

At one time, the submersible pressure gauge (SPG) was a scuba diving option. It is now mandatory equipment required by all U.S. sport scuba diving agencies for any of their sanctioned activities. It is the only way to assess accurately how much air you have to continue the dive. Diving without an SPG is like driving a car without a fuel gauge.

Selecting a Pressure Gauge

The SPG attaches to a high-pressure hose, which is connected to one of the high-pressure ports on the first-stage regulator. Most SPGs are built to withstand hard use, with durable metal housings, rubber protective cases, and consoles all helping to protect the delicate gauge mechanism. A swivel head, large markings, and scratch-resistant glass make an SPG easier to read underwater. Examples of pressure gauges are illustrated in Figs. 4-1 and 4-2.

Using the Pressure Gauge

Fig. 4-3 illustrates the proper technique for turning on the air and reading tank pressure. When you open the tank valve, hold the SPG by the hose or the console, not the gauge itself; never point its face toward yourself or anyone else, just in case the viewing lens accidentally shatters under the forces of the high-pressure air which may have leaked into the gauge housing.

SPGs are calibrated in pounds per square inch (U.S.) or kilograms per square centimeter (metric). When the pressure reads half-way between the initial pressure and zero, the tank will contain one-half the volume of air that was present when the tank was full. This is a straight-forward relationship. The volume of air actually available to the diver and the time it will last will depend on the diver's depth and breathing rate. This relationship of available air to depth is discussed further in Chapter 8.

While submerged, many divers keep their SPG secured, not hanging loose. Some buoyancy compensators even have Velcro straps specifically designed to se-

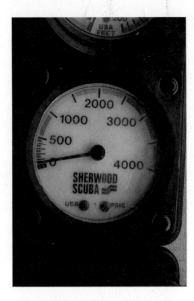

Fig. 4-1 *The submersible pressure gauge is typically a separate instrument or console-mounted device.*

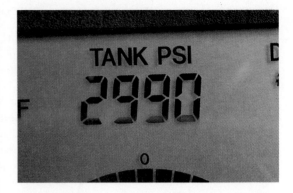

Fig. 4-2 *With the advent of combined-use instrumentation, the tank pressure is but one part of the information being reported to the diver as part of the console's data.*

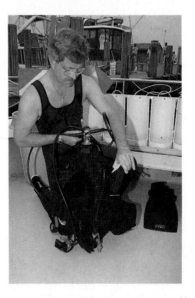

Fig. 4-3 *To avoid injury to yourself or anyone else, hold the gauge away from you and others while turning on the air.*

cure the gauge or console. You can also attach it to a tank strap or tuck it under your BC.

Wherever you secure it, do not forget to use it. Develop the habit of regularly monitoring your gauge to track your air consumption and remaining air supply.

Care and Maintenance of the SPG

Rinse the SPG thoroughly after diving without disconnecting the high-pressure hose from the first-stage regulator. When storing it, do not crimp the hose but keep it straight or in a gentle curve instead.

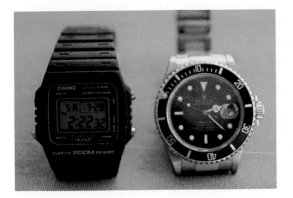

Fig. 4-4 *Two different types of diving watches.*

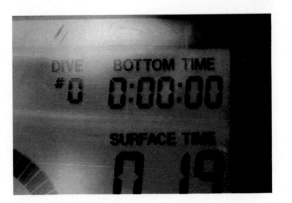

Fig. 4-5 *Some computer consoles are also dive timers.*

UNDERWATER TIMING DEVICES

It is almost impossible to correctly estimate the passage of time underwater because your attention is diverted by other aspects of the dive, such as your buddy, equipment, the environment, and yourself. With so much happening, time passes quickly. Yet elapsed time while diving is a critical factor in your safety and health.

Your time on the bottom, except for the shallowest of dives, must stay within certain limits in order to avoid decompression problems. (See Chapter 9.) Because of this, a timing device, such as one of the watches shown in Fig. 4-4, is necessary equipment for a safe dive.

Selecting a Diving Watch

Not all water-resistant or waterproof watches can withstand increased water pressure without damage. A diving watch should be labeled as pressure tested to at least 220 feet or 67 meters, but 660 feet or 200 meters is preferred for extra strength.

The watch illustrated on the right in Fig. 4-4 has a movable bezel surrounding the watch face, which is used to mark elapsed time. The bezel is tight to the watch to eliminate any accidental movements, once set. A large, serrated edge makes a bezel easier to set, especially when you are wearing gloves. Some watches, like the one pictured on the left of Fig. 4-4, incorporate a liquid crystal display (LCD) stop watch that displays elapsed time at the punch of a button.

Fig. 4-5 shows the timing device built into one of the modern console, multi-function computers now available. These devices, along with some diving watches also available, do not need to be set to begin timing your diving activities, but activate the dive-timing mechanism as soon as your depth in the water exceeds a preset, relatively shallow depth.

In addition to monitoring diving "bottom time," some of the newer timing devices also keep track of your "surface interval," the time that elapses between dives.

DEPTH GAUGE

A diver's depth gauge is the handiest way of monitoring your depth. When you dive, you must know your exact depth to avoid problems with decompression. (See Chapters 9 and 10.) As mentioned, increased depth reduces the air time available for breathing. The effects of the gases in the air also become factors in determining dive times, and vary according to the depth to which you dive. Because of these factors, a depth gauge should go on every dive with you.

Selecting a Depth Gauge

There are four kinds of depth gauges: capillary, bourdon tube, diaphragm, and electronic. Depth gauges are relatively accurate, but can become inaccurate with normal use. Therefore, it is recommended that you have your depth gauge calibration checked periodically.

The capillary gauge is the simplest and least expensive. It has no moving parts and is extremely useful down to about 60 feet. Examination of the depth marks will show you why its readability suffers at greater depths.

"Capillary" refers to the thin plastic tube shown in Fig. 4-6. The depth is read at the point on the dial where air and water meet in the tube. As a diver descends, increased water pressure forces water into the open end of the tube to compress the air trapped inside. At 33 feet (10 meters), for example, the air in the tube is compressed to half its original volume; at 66 feet (20 meters), it is compressed to one-third; at 99 feet (30 meters) to one-fourth, and so on.

If the water section is fragmented by air bubbles, the reading is inaccurate. If air bubbles are forming, it usually means the tube is dirty and should be removed

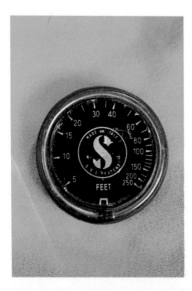

Fig. 4-6 The capillary tube depth gauge is accurate for shallow diving but becomes less easy to read accurately at greater depths.

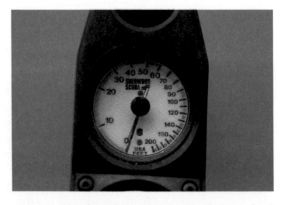

Fig. 4-7 The bourdon tube or diaphragm depth gauges offer greater accuracy below 30 feet.

and cleaned. If you are diving in salt water, salt crystals can form inside the tube but can be removed with a pipe cleaner.

The bourdon tube and diaphragm depth gauges are more expensive than the capillary gauge, but they are easier to read below 30 feet. (See Fig. 4-7.) As you descend, ambient pressure is transmitted to an internal mechanism which, in turn, moves the indicator on the face of the gauge.

The depth gauge shown in Fig. 4-8 incorporates a maximum depth indicator. As you descend, both needles move to show your actual depth. On ascent, the maximum depth needle remains at the deepest depth attained, while the other needle continues to register your present depth. This maximum depth needle eliminates the guesswork of determining your maximum depth after a dive, which is particularly important when monitoring diving depths and times relative to decompression; the needle movement on ascent allows you to monitor ascent rate, an equally important factor in diver safety. Maximum depth indicators must be reset after each dive and care should be taken not to jar the gauge before the reading is taken.

Because of its contribution to diver safety and the minimal increase in expense for it, the maximum depth indicator needle is recommended when a bourdon tube or diaphragm depth gauge is purchased.

An electronic depth gauge, whether it is separate or incorporated into an electronic console, uses a pressure-sensitive input and digital output on an LCD display. It can be extremely accurate and is quite reliable. One is illustrated in Fig. 4-9.

Depth gauges are calibrated in feet of seawater (fsw) in the U.S. system and in meters of seawater (msw) in the metric system. For conversion purposes, 1 foot of sea water equals 0.3 meter and 1 meter of seawater equals 3.3 feet; thus 33 feet equals 10 meters, which equals 1 sea level atmosphere. These factors may be useful if you dive with a gauge marked for a measuring system other than the one you are familiar with.

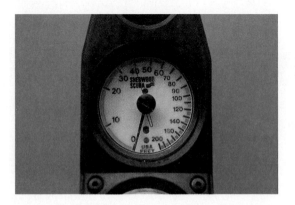

Fig. 4-8 *This depth gauge incorporates a maximum depth indicator needle, which registers that on the most recent dive the maximum dive was 40 feet.*

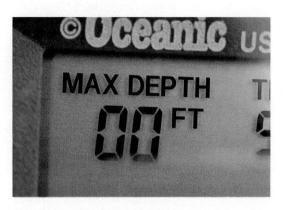

Fig. 4-9 *Electronic depth indicators are accurate and reliable and are incorporated into most dive computers.*

DIVE COMPUTERS

Dive computers (electronic diving monitors) have become popular among sport divers because of their ease of reading and the numerous functions they perform. (See Figs. 4-10 and 4-11.) No instrument, electronic or mechanical, can guarantee against malfunction or misuse errors. The diver must use these tools intelligently and periodically test their accuracy.

As we discuss in Chapter 9, decompression sickness can be avoided if the diver does not absorb excessive nitrogen resulting from breathing compressed air at depth over an extended period of time. Although other factors contribute to decompression sickness, the one major problem has been that sport divers do not always monitor their diving depth and time accurately and do not manipulate that information correctly with the dive tables. The diving computer simplifies this process by both constantly monitoring the diver's depth and time and calculating the diver's status relative to decompression sickness parameters. The principal benefit of the dive computer is that it eliminates the need for dive table manipulations and thereby reduces the possibility of data retrieval and calculation errors on the part of a diver. Other conditions that might make one susceptible to decompression sickness are not monitored by most dive computers and should not be ignored by conscientious divers.

Most dive tables, as we shall see in Chapter 10, assume that a sport dive is "square"—the diver goes straight down, remains at a constant depth, and comes almost straight up at a fixed rate of ascent. Actual sport dives, on the other hand, do not follow a square pattern but follow what is called a multilevel pattern. The com-

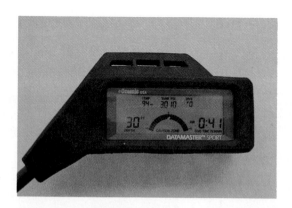

Fig. 4-10 Dive computers today are sometimes incorporated into a multifunction console that monitors many aspects of your diving activity.

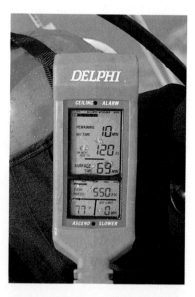

Fig. 4-11 One of the many diving computers now available to the sport scuba diver.

puter follows the multilevel diving pattern of the diver and calculates the diver's decompression sickness exposure.

The use of a dive computer is covered in greater depth in the *Advanced Manual*. A computer is simply an electronic device that constantly computes and compares information derived from an actual dive pattern against the theoretical limits for safe diving. The dive computer is best used as a guide in making decisions to avoid decompression sickness.

Please remember that neither dive tables nor a dive computer can absolutely assure that you will not be struck with decompression sickness. Use both in accordance with the manufacturer's directions and follow a conservative dive plan.

Guidelines for the prudent use of dive computers are as follows:

1. Read the operation manual thoroughly.
2. Each diver should dive with his or her own dive computer.
3. Dive conservatively with respect to the no-decompression limits.
4. Make only no-decompression dives.
5. Do not exceed the computer-specified ascent rate.
6. Make a safety stop at between 10 and 30 feet for 3 to 5 minutes during ascent; many sources recommend that this stop take place at 20 feet.
7. Make your deepest dive first.
8. Avoid repetitive dives in excess of 100 feet.
9. Do not turn the computer off before its outgassing period is complete or if multiday dives are contemplated.
10. Recognize the computer failure indications and abide by failure procedures.
11. Abide by the flying-after-diving procedures.

Some of these rules may not become clear until you complete more training. With the help of your instructor, understand these rules before your first computer-assisted dive.

COMPASS

The compass increases convenience and safety of a dive. It is the easiest way to maintain a valid sense of direction in murky or turbid water where visibility is poor and at night both underwater and on the surface. The compass can also indicate the way to shore. In some coastal waters, it is not uncommon to descend under blue skies and surface in thick fog.

The compass is a valuable navigational tool even when visibility is excellent. Since travel in scuba gear is usually easier below the surface than on it, using a compass allows directed travel there without having to make repeated trips to the surface to check direction.

Selecting a Compass

The simple watchband compass shown in Fig. 4-12 is the least expensive. It gives general direction but is not very accurate. The larger side-reading compass or the top-reading compass is more accurate and gives good directional information.

The top-reading compass shown in Fig. 4-13 is designed for complete underwa-

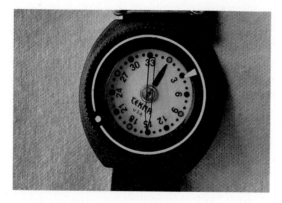

Fig. 4-12 *The watchband compass is the least expensive diving compass but is not very accurate for navigation purposes.*

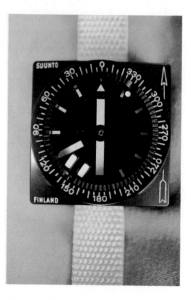

Fig. 4-13 *The top-reading compass is quite accurate and a useful navigational tool.*

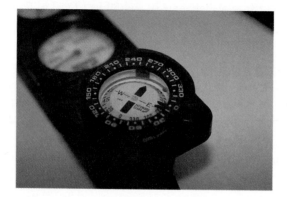

Fig. 4-14 *Similar to the top-reading compass, the side-reading compass is an effective navigational tool.*

ter navigation, and has a movable face marked with desired course bracket lines that can be set for a specific course. The lubber's line provides a sighting line to help maintain a course. The movable face is usually ratcheted, or notched, so it will not move accidentally after setting.

The side-reading compass (Fig. 4-14) is similar to the top-reading compass in features except that the course (discussed below) can be read through the side-reading window.

Compasses may be held in a hand, worn on the wrist, mounted on a console, or mounted on a separate board or slate for use. Remember, compass needles are attracted to ferrous metals such as steel, boats, and wrecks.

Using the Compass

A compass displays direction in terms of a 360° circle, where 0° is north, 90° is east, 180° is south, and 270° is west. To travel any course with a wrist-mounted, top-

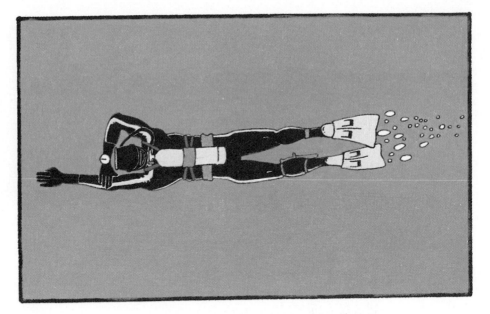

Fig. 4-15 *Using the top-reading compass to maintain a course underwater.*

reading compass, point the arm without the compass straight ahead, then grasp that arm's elbow with your compass hand so the compass is directly ahead of and slightly below your eyes. Your straight arm should be pointing in the direction of travel as shown in Fig. 4-15.

If you want to swim a westerly course, set the movable bracket lines on the face of the compass opposite 270° on the bezel. Then rotate yourself until the compass needle is between the brackets. To maintain the heading, simply keep the compass needle between the bracket lines and sight along the lubber's line and your straight arm. (See Fig. 4-16.)

To travel a course with a side-reading compass, the procedure is similar except that the course you wish is set in the side-reading window. The arm or console, if console mounted, again serves as the pointer for the course of travel. See Fig. 4-17.

Regardless of the type of compass used for navigation, hold the compass level. When tilted too far, the compass card will no longer move freely and will drag on the compass body, preventing accurate direction control.

To gain confidence with compass navigation, practice walking through a few compass courses on dry land.

Reciprocal Dive Courses

Before you can compute a reciprocal dive course (to come back on the same course line you went out on), you must first determine the compass heading for the outbound course. For example, assume the outbound course is 290°. The reciprocal (return or inbound) course is 180° from the outbound course. In this example, it would be computed 290° − 180° = 110°. If the outbound course is less than 180°, the proper procedure is to add 180° instead of subtracting.

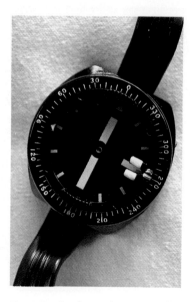

Fig. 4-17 *Maintaining a course of 270° using a side-reading compass.*

Fig. 4-16 *Look at the top-reading compass to maintain a 270° course.*

More advanced compass use and navigation will be learned as your training progresses.

NATURAL NAVIGATION

Although the compass is a valuable piece of equipment, you can also use natural aids to help in underwater navigation. Maintaining your direction and orientation underwater without a compass can be greatly enhanced if you use navigational aids, which are essentially elements of the environment.

Before entering the water, study the diving area from a high vantage point if possible. Since the underwater environment is normally an extension of the shoreline, land contours above the water are indicative of land contours beneath the water. Note the relative location of any kelp beds, shallow reefs, rocks, and other features that can be used later to help establish your location and direction. Information about the speed and direction of any currents is also relevant. The condition of the tides should be considered and verified with appropriate charts and tables. Notice the position of the sun or moon and the direction the light rays enter the water. Anticipate the movement of the sun or moon during your planned dive.

As you descend, maintain your orientation by facing the direction of your initial heading. Pay close attention to your surroundings to note identifiable features.

Check the direction and strength of the current. Kelp and grass lean with the current. Small particulate matter flows with the current. Normally, it is wise to begin your dive into the current and then take advantage of the current as you return to your entry point or the boat. Above all, avoid having to fight the current toward the end of your dive.

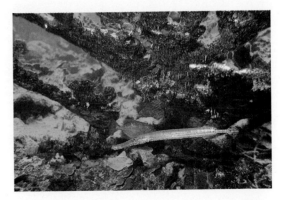

Fig. 4-19 *Fish that tend to hover in the ocean like this trumpetfish will "swing" with the surge. The part of the swing that moves the fish further is toward shore, as this is the strongest part of the surge.*

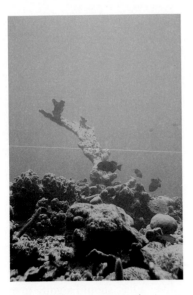

Fig. 4-18 *When diving in the ocean, look for distinctive coral formations for natural navigation landmarks. In fresh water, rock formations can serve the same purpose.*

On the bottom, note any features that can be used as landmarks. Check the bottom contour and depth. Normally, deeper means farther from shore. The ambient light level and presence of various colors are also natural depth indicators.

Throughout the dive, look for features that were observed during your initial overview of the dive area. (See Fig. 4-18.) Use any natural directional indicators that are available such as ripple marks on a sandy bottom, which generally run parallel to the prevailing surface waves. Sand dollars, standing on end, generally run perpendicular to shoreline with exposed tops leaning away from the current. Surge always moves in and out perpendicular to the prevailing waves. The surge toward the shore is always stronger than the surge away from it.

Sometimes a constant sound or noise can be used as a directional indicator, mainly by using the change of intensity of the sound to indicate your movement toward or away from the source. In general, though, sound is virtually impossible to pinpoint directionally under water.

Natural navigation requires a keen awareness of the environment. (See Fig. 4-19.) You can develop it as you continue to experience the underwater environment and exercise your powers of observation. Start by developing the habit of looking back at significant landmarks so you will recognize them more easily on your return. For a complete discussion of underwater navigation techniques, see the *Advanced Manual*.

5 Tools and Accessories

- Float and Flags
- Signalling Devices
- Dive Knife and Dive Tool
- Underwater Light
- Thermometer
- Logbook and Dive Tables
- Spare Parts and Repair Kit
- Gear Bag

At the conclusion of Chapter 5, you will be able to:

1. Explain what the red and white diver's flag should signify to approaching boaters.
2. Explain what the alpha flag means.
3. State the appropriate location for the whistle you should wear when diving.
4. Tell how a day-night flare can attract attention during the day.
5. Describe where you will place the chemical light stick when used during a night dive.
6. Name two properties of a good diving knife or tool.
7. Explain two considerations in the placement of a diving knife or tool.
8. Name two types of light source used in underwater lights.
9. Explain why a thermometer is a useful diving tool.
10. Name at least five of the entries you will make in your dive log following each dive.

KEY TERMS

Sport diver flag	Alpha flag	Chemical glow light
Dive tool	Dive knife	Sheath
Sealed beam	Snorkel keeper	Silicone grease

Special Equipment and Tools

People need special tools for most jobs and recreational activities. A tool may be as simple as a baseball glove or as complicated as a computer, but whatever it is, it makes the task easier and safer. After skin diving and scuba diving began to grow in the 1950s, it did not take long for waterproof and corrosion-resistant tools to be developed. Now, a diver has tools to notify others of his location, to perform underwater tasks, to gather and record information, and to repair and protect equipment. Once you have adapted to the underwater environment, using tools becomes a significant part of diving.

FLOAT AND FLAG

A boater on the surface can rarely see a diver underwater, and many do not recognize diver bubbles. Even when buddy teams are at the surface, they may be difficult to see from a fast-moving boat. A dive flag can help make a diver more visible; that is why it is an important safety tool. It helps reduce the danger to the dive team by warning boats of their presence. Boaters around a dive flag are to stay clear or proceed at very slow speed with a careful watch.

Fig. 5-1 shows the diving flag commonly used, along with its accompanying float. It is red with a white diagonal stripe and means "there are free-swimming divers below; keep well clear at slow speed." It is the primary flag used by divers and is governed by tradition and some state regulations. Learn the regulations for areas where you dive.

Another flag used by divers is the alpha flag which is white and blue with a "V" cut into the outside edge. It is primarily a boater's flag that means "this vessel has divers below and its maneuverability is restricted." It is generally used when divers

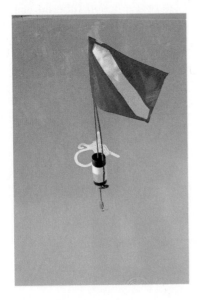

Fig. 5-1 *The sport diver flag and float advises boaters that divers are underwater.*

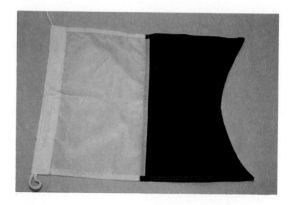

Fig. 5-2 *The alpha flag is typically the flag shown by vessels with divers underwater.*

are tethered to the vessel by hoses or lines, such as during commercial diving operations. The use of the alpha flag is governed by U.S. Coast Guard regulations and applies only to international and inland navigable waterways. Many divers display both flags on their dive boat. The alpha flag is shown in Fig. 5-2. Either flag should be flown only when divers are actually in the water.

WHISTLE (SURFACE SIGNAL)

Your buddy is your constant underwater companion; you should never leave your buddy, and the two of you should not stray far from the boat, dive float, or beach. For those who have strayed or been separated from their buddies accidentally, a whistle is a lot better than a yell on the surface for attracting the attention of buddies or people on boats or on the shore. A simple whistle made of plastic or some other noncorrosive material tied to the oral inflation tube on your buoyancy compensator (Fig. 5-3) is easier to hear over wind and waves and is less tiring than shouting or waving your arms.

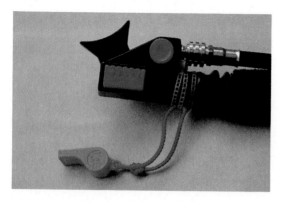

Fig. 5-3 *Emergency diving whistle tied to oral inflator hose of BC.*

FLARE

A special flare, pictured in Fig. 5-4, has a combination of red smoke and a very bright red light, for either day or night use for attracting attention in an emergency. It can be taped to a belt or knife sheath for carrying, and even though it is water-proof, it will not ignite while submerged. Although available in most marine stores, flares are not in common use.

For night diving, the chemical glow light, shown in Fig. 5-5, is an excellent auxiliary light and/or safety device. A small glass container surrounded by a sealed plastic tube, it is activated by simply bending the tube to break the internal glass container. When the two chemicals inside the light stick mix, they create a glow that is readily visible underwater at night. The lights are available to glow in green, blue, or red. A common practice is to tie the light stick to the tank valve. In this position, it will float upright and not interfere with night vision of the diver wearing it.

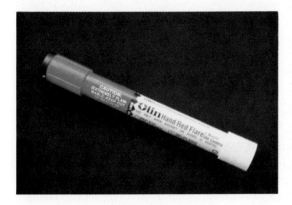

Fig. 5-4 Emergency day and night flare.

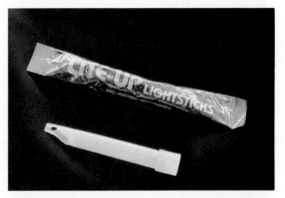

Fig. 5-5 Chemical light sticks come in a variety of sizes and colors for night diving.

They are used on night dives in several different ways. Both buddies should activate their light sticks at the beginning of a night dive to keep track of each other. Dive masters may wear a different color light stick so their divers can locate them easily. Some night dive plans may call for activation of the light stick only if divers become lost or in case of an emergency.

DIVE KNIFE AND DIVE TOOL

A knife is such a multipurpose diving tool that it might be called the diver's primary tool. It can be a hammer, saw, screwdriver, lever, pry bar, ruler, probe, and cutting tool. A primary purpose of a knife is to cut fishing line if entangled; therefore a section of the blade should be sharp enough to cut through monofilament. It is rarely, if ever, used as a weapon against underwater life. Trying to fight off a shark with a knife is not only ridiculous, it could aggravate the situation. A knife or tool should not be used to molest or injure animals or the environment. It can be used in food gathering, collecting, and to assist in underwater work.

The dive knives and dive tools shown in Fig. 5-6 are made of high-quality, non-corrosive steel that is strong enough for prying yet hard enough to hold a sharp edge. The blade piece extends all the way through a guard and into an unbreakable handle for better resistance to breakage at the handle. The hard steel butt at the end of the handle is provided for pounding when using the knife or tool as a hammer.

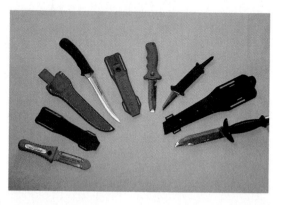

Fig. 5-6 *Various dive knives and dive tools commonly used by sport scuba divers.*

The knife sheath has long, stretchable leg straps, strong buckles, and a strong positive retainer to keep the knife in place. The dive knife sheath covers the blade completely.

For accessibility with both hands and to avoid snagging anything on the handle, the knife is worn by many divers on the inside of the calf, opposite the dominant hand. The same advantage can be gained by mounting it on the console. Some divers prefer just a small line-cutting knife worn on the weight belt or BC. Regardless of size or type, rinse and dry both knife and sheath after every dive. An occasional disassembly, cleaning, sharpening, and oiling will help keep a knife fully functional.

UNDERWATER LIGHT

An underwater light makes seeing many attractions on a night dive possible. It also adds a new dimension to daytime diving. Since most colors are absorbed by water below 60 feet, a diving light restores vivid reds and yellows to the seascape that are lost without light.

There are two types of diving light. The first is basically a standard flashlight with a light bulb that is sealed to be watertight, like those shown in Fig. 5-7. The second light is much brighter because it uses a sealed beam lamp along with more powerful batteries. The sealed beam is like a waterproof automobile headlight with

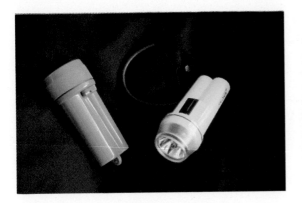

Fig. 5-7 *Typical small underwater lights.*

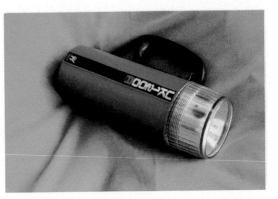

Fig. 5-8 *Larger sealed-beam rechargeable light.*

a built-in reflector and lens. This type of underwater light may also use a rechargeable battery, which lasts from 1 to 3 hours before needing recharging. It is shown in Fig. 5-8.

Batteries without supplied rechargers may have a lower initial cost, but in the long run replacement battery costs may drive the ultimate cost above the cost of the rechargeable variety of light. Today, you can purchase rechargeable batteries of all sizes with rechargers, and this additional investment might be a worthwhile consideration for any underwater light you purchase which is not supplied with a recharger. Dive light technology has advanced to such a degree that very bright lights are available in very compact units if the diver is willing to make the expenditure.

The diving light must be waterproof and pressure proof. It is best to store it with the battery separate from the housing, if possible, to avoid accidental corrosion of the housing. Make sure everything is clean and dry before storage. For a complete discussion of night diving and underwater lights, see the *Advanced Manual*.

THERMOMETER

A waterproof, pressure-proof thermometer, such as the one shown in Fig. 5-9, can be carried on the wrist strap of your watch, attached to a diving slate, or attached to a console. Diving instrument packages often include temperature as one bit of information displayed to the diver on an electronic console, as shown in Fig. 5-10.

Knowing water temperature helps in planning future dives. Temperature readings can also be used to define a thermocline, a change in water temperature with depth, which is discussed in greater detail in Chapter 11.

LOGBOOK AND DIVE TABLES

A logbook is the place to record your diving experiences for the fun of recalling them later and also to give you data for planning future dives more intelligently. The logbook can contain a description of diving sites, depths, visibility, other con-

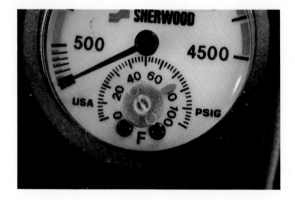

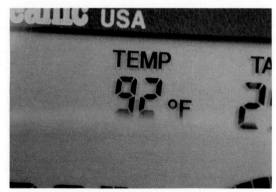

Fig. 5-9 *Waterproof and pressure-proof thermometer.*

Fig. 5-10 *Some electronic consoles also provide temperature information.*

ditions, diving times, and total diving hours plus whatever else you may want to record in it. The diver's logbook is also vital if an emergency occurs, and the dive data it contains is critical to ensure proper medical treatment.

Recording temperatures, for example, helps you evaluate exposure suit needs for dives at the same time the following year.

The data from a previous dive is definitely needed for the planning of a repetitive dive. Having the data recorded helps avoid errors from a faulty memory.

A trend within the diving industry is to require a logbook as well as a certification card as evidence of recent diving experience when you want to rent diving equipment or dive from a dive boat.

An underwater slate can be used to record times, depths, temperatures, and other observations for transfer to the logbook later. A slate can also be used to communicate with your buddy during the dive.

A waterproof set of dive tables is useful for planning on the surface as well as for emergency adjustments to the dive plan underwater should the need arise (Fig. 5-11).

Fig. 5-11 *A diving logbook, a typical waterproof dive table, and several types of dive slates.*

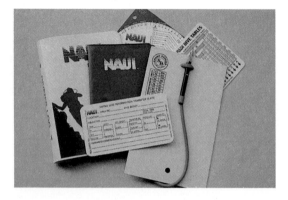

Spare parts and repair kit

Parts

1. Fin strap and buckle
2. Mask strap and buckle
3. Tank "O" rings
4. Regulator mouthpiece
5. Snorkel keeper
6. Regulator high-pressure hose
7. Regulator low-pressure hose

6. Waterproof tape
7. Silicone grease
8. Needle and thread
9. Wet suit cement
10. Nylon line
11. Silicone spray

Expendables

1. Batteries
2. Seasickness medication
3. Antifog solution
4. Sunblock
5. Topical medications

Tools

1. Pliers
2. Adjustable wrench
3. Allen wrench for regulator port plugs
4. Small screwdriver

Note: Any medications only should be carried based upon appropriate medical advice.

SPARE PARTS AND REPAIR KIT

The loss or breakage of a part as simple as a fin strap can end the day's diving. A simple repair kit of tools and spare parts in a dry container can help keep your gear working and you diving (Fig. 5-12). Typical repair kit components are shown in the box above.

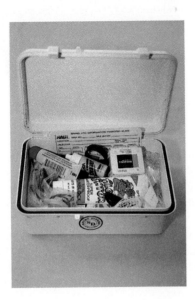

Fig. 5-12 *Sometimes called a "Save-A-Dive" box, this dry box contains the things that a diver might need to make temporary repairs on a given dive.*

GEAR BAG

A gear bag, such as the one shown in Fig. 5-13, is for carrying your gear from place to place and for keeping it somewhat organized. The gear bag you select should be large enough to hold all your gear, except the tank and weight belt. Seams, handles, and zippers should be heavy duty and noncorrosive for durability. Heavy cotton, nylon, canvas, reinforced vinyl, plastic, and Cordura are often used for gear bags. Handles should be connected to straps which go completely around the bag.

When packing your gear bag, put fins, boots, gloves, knives, and other nonbreakable items on the bottom. Pack more delicate items such as masks, regulators, instruments, and cameras in separate rigid containers for extra protection. Tanks are usually carried separately. Weight belts should always be handled separately for safety. Wet items should not be stored in your gear bag unless it is designed to allow water to drain out and the gear to dry.

Exposure suits are best allowed to dry outside the gear bag in any case, to prevent mildew and odors from building up. When you are diving on a boat, it is common courtesy and smart to keep all of your loose diving equipment in the bag except when you are in the water wearing it.

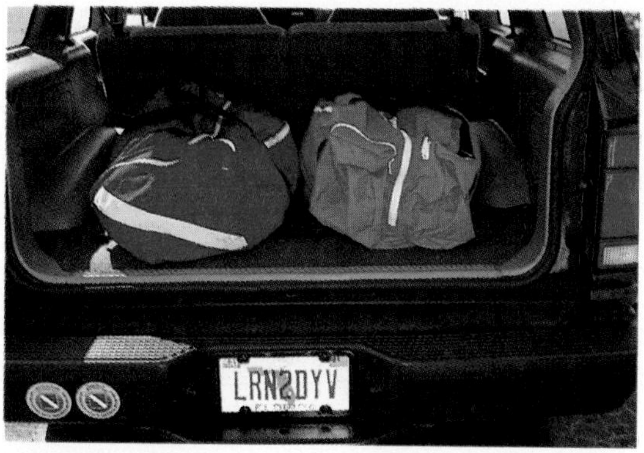

Fig. 5-13 *One of many varieties of gear bags available to the scuba diver.*

SUMMARY

The amazing growth of diving as a sport depended almost entirely on the development of diving equipment. It has enabled thousands of swimmers to experience the underwater world with comfort and freedom. Continuing advances in diving equipment are enabling divers to operate more efficiently and comfortably in and on the water.

The future of diving will be exciting, but so is the present. Diving equipment developed in the last three decades has solved dozens of problems humans encountered when entering the underwater world. The future undoubtedly holds more of the same kind of progress for even better times in inner space.

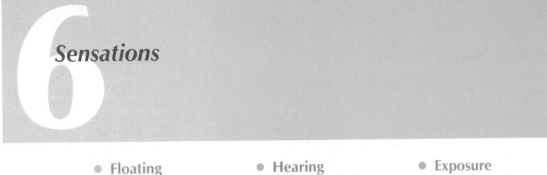

6 Sensations

- Floating
- Seeing
- Hearing
- Hand Signals
- Exposure

At the conclusion of Chapter 6, you will be able to:

1. Explain the concept of buoyancy.

2. Describe the different types of buoyancy.

3. Tell how much air the fully inflated adult lungs contain.

4. State the weight of 1 cubic foot of sea water.

5. Explain why objects underwater appear to be closer and larger than they do above the water.

6. Taking the colors blue, orange, yellow, red, and green, tell the order in which these colors seem to disappear in the water.

7. State how much faster sound moves underwater.

8. Explain why it is virtually impossible to determine the direction of sound underwater.

9. Demonstrate the hand signals for OK; stop; danger; low on air; out of air; I want to share air; going up; going down; buddy up.

10. Tell how much faster heat is lost in water than in air.

KEY TERMS

Buoyancy	Negative buoyancy	Archimedes
Displacement	Refraction	Turbidity
Absorption	Conduction	Evaporation

Floating, Seeing, Hearing, and Exposure

Entering even shallow water bombards you with new sensations. You see, hear, smell, taste, and feel differently in water than in air. To really grasp these differences, it helps to know what water is and how it differs from air. This knowledge will help explain the various sensations and how to adapt to them.

FLOATING

The feeling of buoyancy, or being pushed upward by water, is perhaps the most relaxing and pleasant of all the underwater sensations. The buoyancy we feel in water gives most of us the only relief we will ever know from the constant downward pull of gravity. It is buoyancy that can give a diver almost complete freedom of movement in the vertical dimension.

"Weightless" is a good word for floating, because, if a floating person were to stand on a scale under water, he or she would weigh essentially nothing. Although the individual may not float like a cork, he or she would not sink like a rock either. The reason for this is that approximately 60 percent of the human body is water. Substances either slightly heavier or lighter than water make up the rest of the body. Fat, for example, is not as heavy as muscle. Thus, to put a person into water is like placing a container of water into water—either it sinks very slowly or not at all.

BUOYANCY

Buoyancy is an important condition for divers to control. We know that many people float easily without donning equipment; that is, they have *positive buoyancy*. Some others are *negatively buoyant*: they tend to sink, while others are about *neutrally buoyant*, neither floating nor sinking—they can hang in the water wherever they are.

Why do some people float and others sink? People whose bodies are lighter than the same volume of water float, while those who are heavier sink. The same applies to any material.

For example, a gallon of water weighs about 8.8 pounds, while a gallon of air weighs only one-sixth of an ounce, so a container filled with air floats in water. Similar volumes of wood and foam neoprene are also lighter than water and are therefore positively buoyant. Additionally, since wood is less dense than water and more dense than neoprene, it floats less than the neoprene. Similar volumes of lead, aluminum, and steel, on the other hand, are heavier than water so they sink at speeds which vary with their density.

Controlling Buoyancy

Fortunately for divers and swimmers, the human body has a built-in air chamber that allows control of buoyancy in the water. The lungs hold about 1½ gallons (5 to 6 liters) of air when you inhale completely. This gives your body approximately 10 pounds of *buoyant force* in the water. In other words, 1½ gallons of air will support

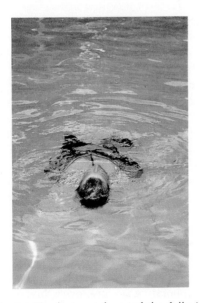

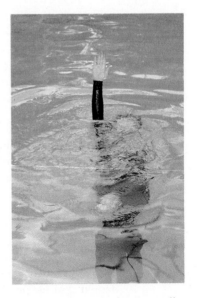

Fig. 6-1 The buoyant force of the fully in- flated lungs.

Fig. 6-2 The negatively buoyant effect of simply raising your arms is demonstrated here, when previously, simply inflating the lungs was enough to keep this person afloat.

about 10 pounds above the surface of the water. During full inhalation, most humans have more than enough buoyancy to lift their eyes and nose out of the water, as shown in Fig. 6-1.

By controlling the amount of air in the lungs, a diver can stay buoyant and relaxed at the surface without getting at all tired. Remember, though, that the normal buoyancy of your body will support only a bit of your body above water. When resting on the surface, do not try to lift your head, shoulders, and arms out of the water because their weight will make you sink. When floating on the surface, stay as low as possible and keep your lungs as full as possible for maximum buoyancy. Fig. 6-2 illustrates the negatively buoyant effect of simply raising both arms above the water.

An individual's buoyancy varies with several factors, including, among others, body build, muscle-fat composition, and lung size. Fat is not as heavy as muscle and bone, so overweight people usually float better than thin people. There are people who cannot float even with proper techniques because their weight is greater than the water they displace. Very thin people cannot float without aids.

Changes in Buoyancy

Another thing that affects buoyancy is the density of water. Salt water, for example, is more dense than fresh water because it contains dissolved salts. The more dense a liquid, the more weight it will support, or the greater its buoyant force. This is why it is easier to float in salt water than in fresh water.

The laws of buoyancy were discovered by Archimedes. He found that the amount of buoyancy an object has depends on the weight of the water it displaces, or pushes away.

To illustrate: If you put a box that measures 12 inches on each side (a volume of 1 cubic foot) into seawater it will displace 64 pounds of seawater and the box will be buoyed up by a force of 64 pounds. This is not to say that the box will float. The box will float only if it weighs *less* than 64 pounds. If the box weighs more than 64 pounds, it will sink. If it weighs exactly 64 pounds, it will neither float nor sink; it will be neutrally buoyant. Thus buoyancy is determined by *both weight and volume*. This is why wet suits and buoyancy compensators increase a diver's buoyancy. They add very little weight while increasing the diver's volume, or displacement.

SEEING

The first time you opened your eyes under water without a mask was probably not only uncomfortable but also disappointing. The feeling of water directly against the delicate tissues of your eyes was probably unpleasant, especially if the water contained chlorine or salt. And disappointing because everything was blurry and out of focus. Most of us get used to the feeling of water, but the blurriness remains because of the way light travels in water and air.

Light

The outer covering of the eye, when surrounded by air, can bend the light, striking it at the exact angle necessary to focus it clearly on the back of the eye. When light enters the eye directly from water, it must be bent at a greater angle to focus at the correct point. Both concepts are illustrated in Fig. 6-3. Unfortunately, the eye is not able to adapt to bend the entering light far enough to focus the rays. Fortunately, we have found a fairly simple solution to obtaining clear vision underwater.

Seeing with a Mask

In theory, a special set of eyeglasses with the right lenses could correct the visual problem, but it turns out that a simple face mask is a much more practical solution. The mask puts an air space in front of your eyes to restore clear vision. In fact, it actually improves underwater vision by providing a slight magnification.

While looking forward, most objects underwater appear approximately 25 percent bigger and 25 percent closer than they really are. Because of the relationship between angle of refraction and viewing angle, objects in the peripheral visual field may be magnified more. The reason for the magnifying effect of the mask is shown in Fig. 6-4. Light transmitted from objects seen travels through the water, through the glass, into the air space behind the glass, and finally into the eye. Since the water, glass, and air all bend the light to different degrees, the light is refracted, or bent, twice instead of only once, as it would be in air only. It is this double bending of the light that causes magnification and actually improves visual images underwater.

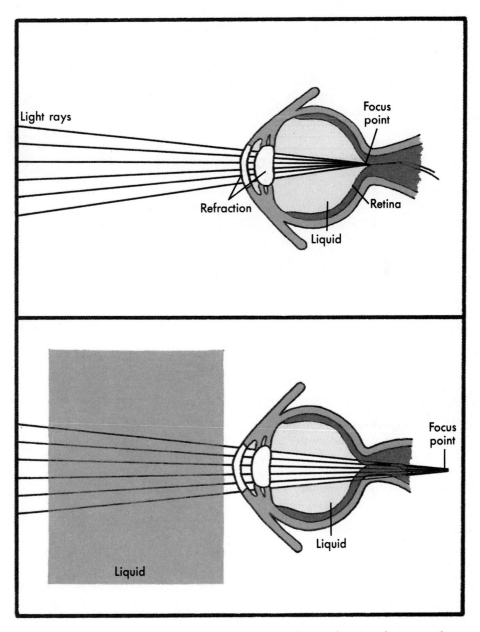

Fig. 6-3 *Seeing on land and in water—the difference in refraction between the two mediums.*

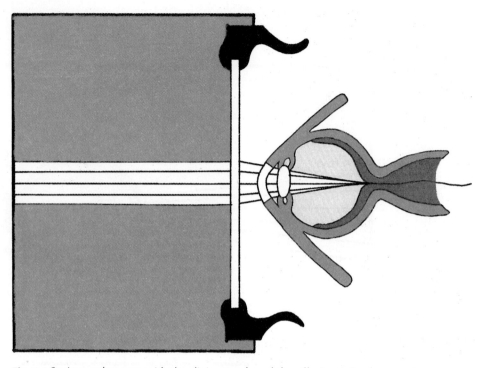

Fig. 6-4 *Seeing underwater with the diving mask and the effect on visual perception.*

Turbidity

Even though your underwater vision improves somewhat, light does not move as well underwater as it does in air. Light from the sun or from artificial lights is scattered or absorbed by particles suspended in the water. Water that contains particles is said to be turbid. Extremely turbid water can almost eliminate visibility and is not normally attractive to many divers. Limited visibility diving is discussed in greater detail in the *Advanced Manual*.

Color

Even if the water is very clear and clean, it still absorbs light. Sunlight is a mixture of colors. Water absorbs colors at different rates. The chart in Fig. 6-5 illustrates in very simple form the absorption of colors in the water. Reds and oranges begin to be absorbed in the first 30 feet. Yellows and greens disappear at around 60 feet, so below this depth, everything goes from a bluish color to completely gray.

Artificial lights used for vision or photography will restore the natural colors no matter what the depth. This concept was mentioned in our previous discussion of underwater lights in Chapter 5, and the use of lights for photography is discussed in the *Advanced Manual*.

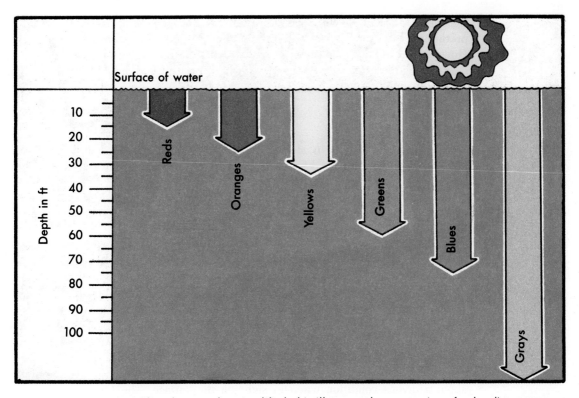

Fig. 6-5 *Though somewhat simplified, this illustrates the progression of color disappearance in water.*

HEARING AND SPEAKING

Sound moves about four times faster under water than in air, but this does not improve your hearing. Ordinary speech is all but impossible below the surface, and it is very difficult to judge the direction of underwater sounds.

In spite of this, the underwater world can be a noisy place. You can hear equipment clanking together, motorboats buzzing at the surface, bubbles leaving your regulator and other regulators, marine life, movement of rocks, churning water, and even raindrops on the surface. But you cannot effectively understand words spoken in water or determine the direction from which sound comes.

The reason you cannot hear voices clearly under water is that sound does not travel well from air to water, or from water to air. You can speak under water, but almost all the sound energy stays in your neck and mouth.

You cannot determine the direction from which sound is coming because it travels so fast. Your brain determines the direction of a sound by judging the time delay between the arrival of the sound at each ear. In air, sounds coming from your right hit your right ear first, then your left ear, and your brain is capable of interpreting this tiny time delay to determine that the sound is coming from the right. However, in water, since sound moves so much faster, the brain is not capable of interpreting the briefer time interval, so when you hear a sound under the water, it seems to come from all around.

HAND SIGNALS

Since talking underwater is almost impossible, the diving community has developed a set of standard hand signals to meet the need for underwater communication.

As there may sometimes be local or regional variations of the signals illustrated in this manual, they should be reviewed with your buddy before diving so that you both agree on the meanings to avoid confusion underwater.

Figs. 6-6 to 6-9 indicate how a diver "says" OK both under and on the surface. Figs. 6-10 to 6-19 show other common diving hand signals. These signals are used extensively by divers. In a buddy team they are used to monitor the buddy's condition routinely, and to encourage an anxious diver to relax and enjoy the dive. Generally, if your buddy shows you an OK sign, you should return it with a like sign if you too are OK, or give him or her whatever sign is appropriate to describe your problem. After entering the water from a dive boat, turn toward the dive boat, and signal OK if everything is under control and you are ready to go. In boat or beach diving, the two-arm OK sign is the way for the boat/beach master to inquire about a diver's condition when in sight on the surface. The OK sign should be given toward the boat/beach master if you are in control when you surface at the end of a dive.

You have now reviewed the standard sport diving safety signals plus a few others. Review them again with your buddy and all other divers in your dive group before any dives, especially when there is a diver new to your group who needs to understand any signals that will be used.

EXPOSURE

Most of us would agree that cool water takes your breath away when you enter it, either quickly or slowly. The colder the water, the more unpleasant that sensation is. Very cold water is not only unpleasant, it is also downright dangerous because even short exposures can cause unconsciousness and death. (See Appendix, "Water Temperature Protection Chart.")

Maintaining Body Temperature

On land, the human body has the amazing ability to maintain a core temperature of approximately 98.6° F while temperatures around the body vary widely on the thermometer. The body can be thought of as a living heat machine which generates heat constantly and controls its own temperature by regulating how much of that heat escapes into the surrounding air. The body's heat control system works well in

Text continued on p. 113.

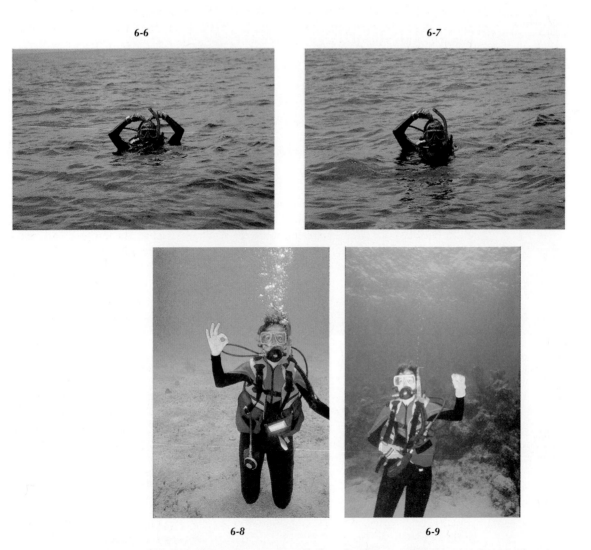

6-6

6-7

6-8

6-9

Fig. 6-6 *OK! OK? This is the signal used when the diver is some distance from the beach or boat and the diver wants the receiver of the hand signal to see and understand the signal clearly.*

Fig. 6-7 *OK! OK? Indication that all is all right using only one arm. This signal is used when the signals below might not be visible due to distance or reduced visibility.*

Fig. 6-8 *OK! OK? The most common and handiest of the OK signals means either "I'm OK" or asks the question "Are you OK?"*

Fig. 6-9 *OK! OK? Signal used to indicate OK when wearing bulky gloves or mittens. This is also the OK sign that is best used in parts of the world where the standard OK hand signal is offensive.*

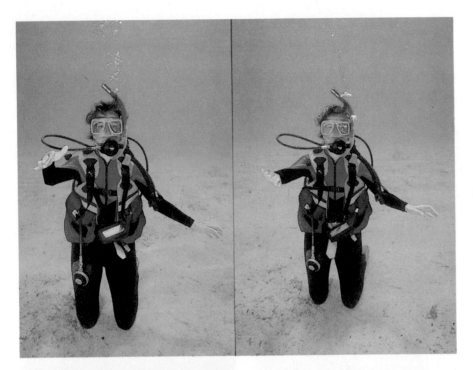

6-10

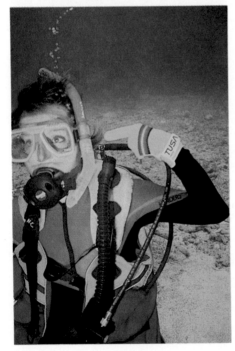

6-11

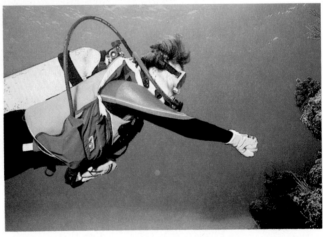

6-12

Fig. 6-10 Something is wrong or not OK. The hand extended outward, palm down, then rocked around the arm's axis indicates that the signaling diver has a minor problem.

Fig. 6-11 A pointing index finger means to look at and when used in conjunction with the not OK hand signal, means that the ear is the problem—usually an ear clearing problem.

Fig. 6-12 Danger! The closed fist aimed at an object or area indicates that it presents a danger to the divers and should be avoided or carefully observed.

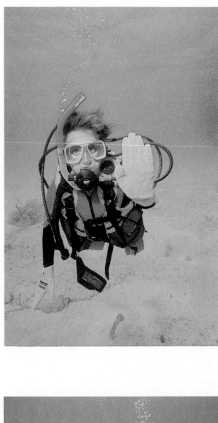

Fig. 6-13 Stop! *This signal is given by your buddy or dive master to indicate that you should stop. On the other hand, it might just be a signal to stay put for a while.*

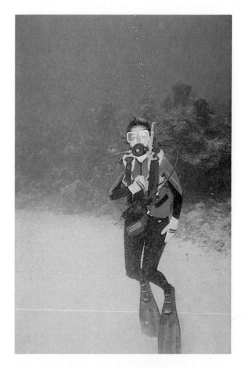

Fig. 6-14 Low on air! *A clenched fist pounding gently on a diver's chest indicates that the diver's air is low.*

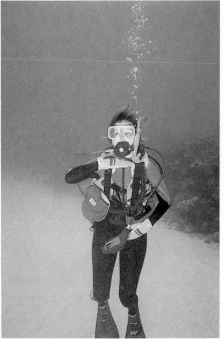

Fig. 6-15 Out of air! *A throat-slashing motion with a hand indicates that the diver has run out of air or cannot breathe through the regulator. It should be followed quickly by the signal below or the diver's ascent.*

Fig. 6-16 I want to share your air! *This signal requests that you offer your octopus, separate alternate air source, or primary regulator for sharing air. If the sharing of air is an emergency, you both should get the situation under control, then ascend to the surface slowly.*

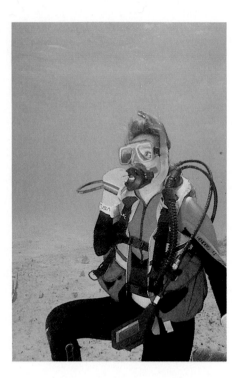

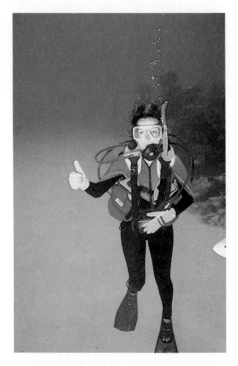

Fig. 6-17 Go up or going up. *Pointing a thumb up tells another diver to go up or that you are going up. A more agitated signal means to hurry.*

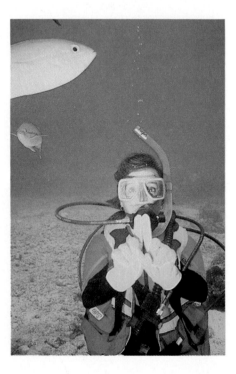

Fig. 6-18 Buddy-up! *Bringing the index fingers of your hands together, is given by your dive master or buddy and means to either get with or stay closer to your buddy.*

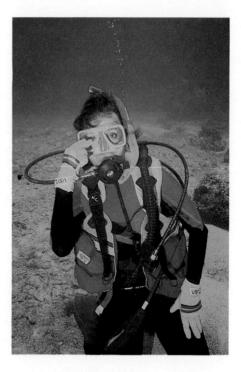

Fig. 6-19 Watch *or* watch me. *Again, pointing an index finger means* look at *whatever is being pointed at.*

air, but because heat is lost to water at a rate about 25 times greater than in air, our heat generation capability is simply not great enough to keep us warm in water.

Conduction and Evaporation

Heat leaves your body in several ways, the two most important being conduction and evaporation.

Conduction refers to heat passing from one medium into another by direct contact. For example, your hand is cold after you hold an ice cube because body heat lost was conducted into the ice cube.

Evaporation occurs when a liquid changes into gas because it has absorbed heat. When you sweat, for example, perspiration absorbs heat as it evaporates to cool your body. This also explains why, after you have been diving and are wet, a gentle breeze can make you quite chilly because heat from your body is absorbed by the water as it evaporates.

Evaporation does not work in the water, but conduction works very well at pulling heat out of your body at a rate 25 times greater than heat loss in air of the same temperature. Conduction explains why even relatively warm water feels cold when you first jump into it. Conduction explains also why we can be comfortable in a 65° room yet cold in a 65° pool. Expressed another way, a 1-hour dive in 65° water would produce heat loss equivalent to standing naked for 25 hours in 65° air.

Maintaining Warmth

Your body, however, does not give up all that heat without a fight. Swimmers often talk about diving into "cold" water and then getting "used to it." What really happens is that a change takes place in your body to slow the conduction of heat into the water. The tiny blood vessels on the surface of the skin constrict automatically when plunged into cold water, to reduce the amount of warm blood that flows to the cold surface of the body. As a result, less heat reaches the skin to be conducted away.

If the reduced blood flow to the skin fails to keep the body warm, and if exercise is not generating enough heat to stay warm, the body core temperature will drop and make the body start shivering. Shivering takes muscular effort, which generates heat to keep warm. An extremely active diver stays warmer than a diver at rest because of the heat generated by muscle activity. Physical activity can produce so much heat, in fact, that a diver in water warmer than 85° F (30° C) may have problems with *over*heating. Cold, however, is a much more common problem for divers.

Effects of Cold Water

The wet or dry suit insulates the diver from the chilling effect of water by surrounding the body with a layer of air or gas bubbles, which reduces the rate at which heat passes from the body into the water. But even with wet or dry suit protection, heat loss still occurs, primarily through the head, neck, and thorax. When heat loss is extreme, mental and motor function can be adversely affected, leading to a loss of strength, difficulty in handling equipment, muscle cramps, and a decrease in problem-solving ability. These are some of the symptoms of hypothermia, a life-threatening condition.

Though mild shivering may begin quite early in a cold water dive, if you ever start shivering violently underwater, terminate the dive. Your body is telling you that its core temperature has dropped significantly. When the body core temperature has dropped to a temperature of about 95° F (35° C), it is known as mild generalized hypothermia. At this temperature, breathing is regular to slightly depressed, there is lack of coordination, the victim begins to feel sleepy, and shivering is usually present. If core temperature drops below about 91.4° F (33° C), shivering typically stops and the diver's level of consciousness diminishes, the heartbeat may become irregular, and myriad other symptoms and signs may develop that indicate potentially lethal problems if the heat loss process is not stopped and reversed immediately.

People have the ability to adapt to harsh environments such that they may tolerate moderate temperature changes approximating 0.5° C. A good precaution for many problems encountered in diving, including both hyper- and hypothermia, is the maintenance of adequate fluid balance. Both hyperthermia and hypothermia are progressive conditions, so be aware of the early signs and symptoms.

Sunburn

Exposure suits can protect you from both cold water and sun exposure. If you snorkel at the surface in warm water without protection, at least to the degree provided by dive skins, you are bombarded by the sun's ultraviolet rays on a sunny day or even a slightly overcast day. Cool water washing over your back and legs makes you unaware that they are actually becoming sunburned.

Sunburn can cause first- and second-degree burns, with some sunburn victims requiring hospitalization. Be careful to limit your exposure to the sun. If you do a lot of snorkeling at the surface of water too warm for wet suits, wear dive skins, a T-shirt and pants or long shorts, or at least water-resistant sunblock.

Hyperthermia, which may sometimes accompany excessive exposure to the sun, may result in additional complications of dehydration, heat exhaustion, and heat stroke—a life-threatening condition.

SUMMARY

No other environment has a more profound effect on the body's five senses than the underwater environment. It changes your seeing, hearing, feeling, tasting, and smelling from normal. It creates a totally different set of experiences which can be thrilling. Some sensations underwater are enjoyable, others require adjustment by special techniques or equipment. In any case, there is no reason for underwater sensations to be unpleasant or uncomfortable.

Thanks to the development of sport diving, your underwater sensations can be pleasant and comfortable. Relish them by learning all you can about the sports of skin and scuba diving, then applying that knowledge.

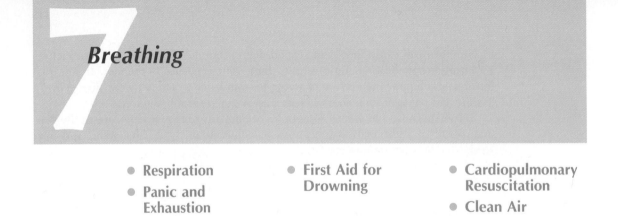

Breathing

- Respiration
- Panic and Exhaustion
- First Aid for Drowning
- Cardiopulmonary Resuscitation
- Clean Air

At the conclusion of Chapter 7, you will be able to:

1. Define the surface area of the respiratory membrane made of alveoli in the lungs.
2. Name the place at which gas exchange takes place in the body.
3. Explain how inhalation and exhalation take place.
4. State the percentages of oxygen and nitrogen contained in the air.
5. Explain why gas presence in the blood controls breathing rate.
6. Describe controlled hyperventilation as it relates to free diving.
7. State how to deal with an anxious feeling during a dive.
8. State the steps in properly performed CPR.
9. Describe in your own terms what "clean air" means.
10. State what type of lubricant is used on scuba gear.

KEY TERMS

Alveoli	Capillaries	Diaphragm
Tidal volume	Vital capacity	Residual volume
Dead-air space	Carbon dioxide	Hypoxia
Panic	CPR	Carbon monoxide

Respiration, Panic and Exhaustion, Resuscitation, Clean Air

Breathing is one habit that we ignore most of the time. We breathe constantly, day and night, without giving it a thought. Swimming or diving under water, however, changes our perception of breathing; the beginning swimmer quickly realizes that he or she cannot "breathe water." Since diving can change, stop, slow down, or speed up the breathing process, let us examine what is going on in your body and mind when you breathe, both on land and in the water.

THE RESPIRATION PROCESS

Respiration refers not only to the simple act of inhaling and exhaling air, but also to the more complex process of exchanging gasses, making energy, and eliminating waste in order to keep the cells of all living creatures alive. Respiration, then, is a primary life process, a process that involves more than the lungs. The circulatory system, including the heart, blood, and vessels, and every living cell in the body are intimately connected with respiration.

The Respiratory System

The center of the human respiratory system is built something like a spongy, up-side down tree, as shown in Fig. 7-1. At the trunk of the upside down tree is the trachea (windpipe), a hollow tube about 4½ inches long and 1 inch wide. The trachea divides into two smaller branches called bronchi, which continue to subdivide into smaller and smaller branches. The smallest twigs, or ducts, end in tiny clusters of air sacs called alveoli. Each cluster looks like a tiny bunch of grapes.

The alveoli are the leaves of the tree. They are extremely thin membranes through which oxygen, carbon dioxide, and other gases pass into and out of the bloodstream. The lungs contain about 300 million alveoli. All of them make up a respiratory membrane with a surface area of about 1,100 square feet, about the surface area of a tennis court!

Each alveolus is surrounded by a network of tiny blood vessels called capillaries. It is at this contact between the respiratory membrane and the capillaries that the gas exchanges in the body actually take place. The inset in Fig. 7-1 illustrates the structure of the alveolus and the terminal duct entering the alveolus as well as the capillaries surrounding the alveolus.

The lungs are protected above, around the sides, and in back by the shoulder girdle, rib cage, and spine. The diaphragm beneath the lungs is a powerful sheet of muscle. When these muscles contract, the diaphragm moves downward and the muscles of the rib cage tend to lift the ribs up and out at the same time. Together, the action of the diaphragm and rib cage increases the volume of the chest cavity. When the volume increases, the pressure within the cavity momentarily decreases and draws air into the lungs through the trachea and bronchi to balance the inside and outside pressures. This process takes place when you inhale.

When the muscles involved in this process relax, the pressure inside momentarily goes up. Since the alveoli are elastic, the air sacs have a tendency to collapse in response to this increased pressure, and air leaves the lungs. This process takes

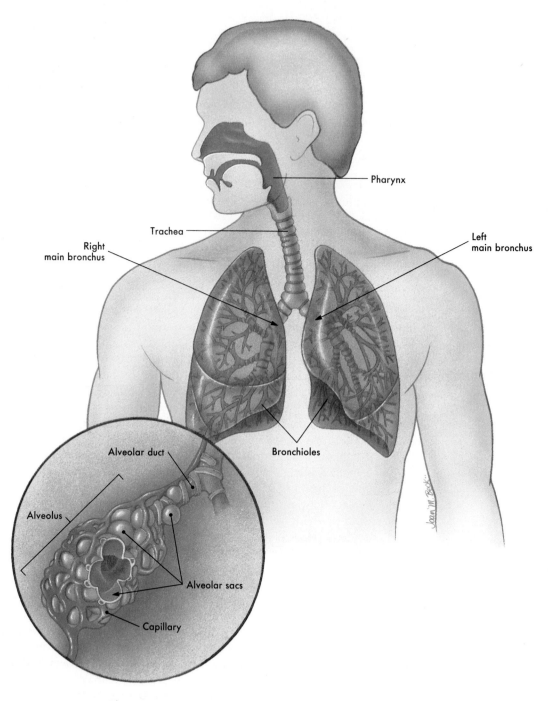

Fig. 7-1 *The respiratory tree and a close look at the alveoli. (From Thibodeau GA and Anthony CP: Structure and function of the body, ed 8, St Louis, 1988, CV Mosby.)*

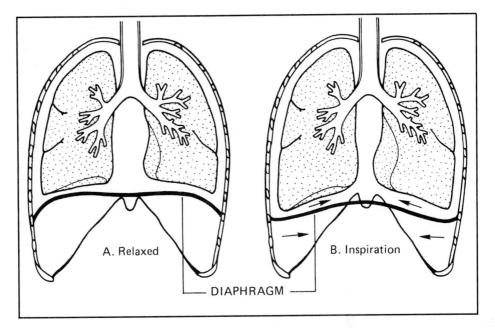

Fig. 7-2 *The relationship of the chest cavity and the diaphragm during the processes of inhaling and exhaling. (From Martin DE: Respiratory anatomy and physiology, St Louis, 1988, CV Mosby.)*

place when we exhale. Fig. 7-2 illustrates the relative position of the diaphragm and rib cage when we inhale and exhale.

Ordinarily, this alternating contraction and relaxation of the muscles involved in breathing takes place automatically. An average adult breathes between 12 and 20 times a minute. Small people and children usually breathe more often, as does an adult who is exercising.

Lung Volumes

An average pair of lungs holds a total volume of 1.5 to 1.6 gallons (5.7 to 6.2 liters) of air. At rest, however, you inhale and exhale only a small fraction of this amount—a little over a pint (0.5 liter). This is called tidal volume, as shown in Fig. 7-3.

Breathing the relatively small tidal volume of air is enough for a person sitting quietly in a chair reading a book, but the long-distance runner or the hard-working diver needs much more air. For example, after inhaling a pint of air during an ordinary breath, you can continue to inhale over 3 quarts (3.3 liters) more. After you exhale the pint of air during an ordinary breath, you can continue exhaling almost 1 additional quart (1 liter).

When you breathe as hard as you can, you move over a gallon (approximately 4.8 liters in young men) of air in one breath. This amount is the vital capacity and it varies a great deal depending upon the size and physical condition of each person.

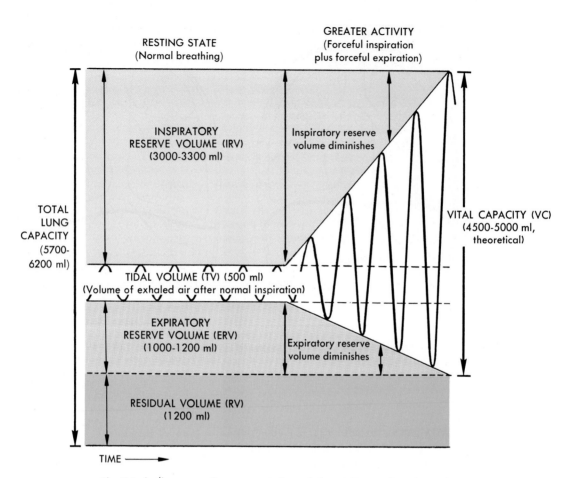

TIME ⟶

Fig. 7-3 *A diagrammatic representation of the various volumes involved in the respiratory process. (From Thibodeau GA and Anthony CP: Structure and function of the body, ed 8, St Louis, 1988, CV Mosby.)*

A small person may have a vital capacity of only 3 quarts (2.8 liters) and a large trained athlete could have one larger than 6 quarts (6.5 liters).

No matter how hard you exhale, you still cannot force all of the air out of your lungs. Over 1 quart (1.2 liters) of air remains in your lungs all the time. This is called residual volume.

All the air you inhale, even during a very large breath, does not find its way to the lungs. Some of it, about a third of a pint (0.16 liter), is in the trachea, throat, and nose, and is exhaled without ever touching the alveoli. This space is called the dead-air space because no gas exchange takes place inside it.

GAS EXCHANGE

The air you inhale is a mixture of about 78 percent nitrogen, 21 percent oxygen, and 1 percent carbon dioxide and other gases. Nitrogen has very little effect on ordinary respiration. It is an inert (chemically inactive) gas that does not support life but has an intoxicating effect under pressure. (See Chapter 9.) Oxygen and carbon dioxide are two gasses that are exchanged during respiration.

The air you exhale has about the same amount of nitrogen, but the oxygen decreases from 21 percent to about 16 percent, and the carbon dioxide increases from 0.03 percent to about 5.6 percent. The body has obviously produced an amount of carbon dioxide roughly equal to the amount of oxygen it absorbs. By maintaining this continuous exchange of gases, the blood and cells of the body maintain sufficient oxygen to support life and prevent an excessive build-up of carbon dioxide, which is unhealthy.

Because the body constantly uses oxygen and produces carbon dioxide, the levels of these two gases in the blood are always changing. When the carbon dioxide in the blood rises, the respiratory center in the brain sends out more frequent impulses, stimulating the diaphragm and chest muscles to contract more frequently and causing you to breathe more rapidly. As the carbon dioxide level in the blood falls, the stimulating action of the respiratory center slows and the breathing rate diminishes. Increasing and decreasing your breathing rate takes place automatically in your body.

Changing the Breathing Rhythm

You can consciously override your breathing rhythm, which is usually automatic and involuntary. For example, talking and holding your breath are two of the many ways to change your breathing rate, all of which affect the exchange of oxygen and carbon dioxide. Changing your breathing rhythm is harmless as long as the balance of gas exchange stays within certain limits. But too much of certain gases or too little of others can cause problems.

Too Much Carbon Dioxide and Too Little Oxygen

There are several factors or practices in sport diving which tend to upset the normal breathing process and can lead to a build-up of carbon dioxide in the blood. At the end of the exhalation phase, the air exhaled into the dead-air space has a high level of carbon dioxide. When you start inhaling, this amount of high carbon dioxide air is inhaled first. Since the natural dead-air space is so small, the carbon dioxide never climbs to any significant level. However, an extremely long or large snorkel can double or triple your dead-air space. If you do not breathe deeper to mix more fresh air with the dead air, carbon dioxide levels in the blood will climb and you will probably have a headache at the end of the dive.

Similarly, a snorkel or regulator with a lot of breathing resistance requires more effort to breathe through. The increased work to breathe produces more carbon dioxide, perhaps more than the body can give off, so the carbon dioxide level in the blood builds up.

Most of us have experienced carbon dioxide excess from swimming or running fast. The "out-of-breath" feeling comes from the respiratory center working overtime in response to the excess carbon dioxide in the blood. This shortness of breath and fatigue on land is not much of a problem, but under water it can be frightening. If you feel "hungry" for air, tired, or weak from working hard while diving, immediately stop, rest, and breathe deeply until you have lost the feeling of air "hunger"—not taking these steps might lead to unconsciousness.

"Skip breathing," a technique that divers once thought would conserve air, can lead to air hunger. Instead of breathing regularly, a diver skips every other breath by holding the breath for the time of a normal inhalation/exhalation. Skip breathing apparently uses only one-half the amount of air, but it really leads to a build-up of carbon dioxide, which ultimately leads to a greater than normal breathing rate. Since it does not work and it is dangerous because of the breath holding, avoid skip breathing while using scuba. Long, slow, steady inhalation and exhalation will minimize breathing effort and is not to be confused with skip breathing where the breath is held.

Many factors that hinder or slow down the exchange of gases not only cause a build-up of carbon dioxide, but also cause a decrease in the amount of oxygen coming into the body during breathing. This oxygen deficiency is called hypoxia. Whether it comes from an equipment breakdown or improper breathing, the signs and symptoms of hypoxia are the same.

Hypoxia can cause heavy breathing, headache, and unconsciousness, just as carbon dioxide build-up does. Hypoxia can also cause nausea, while carbon dioxide excess can cause muscular cramps and fatigue. The treatment for both is increased ventilation of the lungs to restore normal gas exchange levels in the body. Serious cases require taking the diver to the surface for the administration of 100 percent oxygen, which is discussed in the *Advanced Manual*.

Controlled Hyperventilation

Breath-hold divers have been using hyperventilation (fast breathing) for years to help them stay underwater longer. By inhaling completely and exhaling completely three or four times quickly, you can blow off (reduce blood level) carbon dioxide before surface diving. This lets you begin a breath-hold dive with very low carbon dioxide levels in the alveoli and, since the respiratory center in the brain is stimulated to breathe by a high carbon dioxide level, you will not feel the need to breathe as soon after hyperventilation as you would without it.

Hyperventilation, to be free of significant hazard, must be very carefully controlled. Never hyperventilate more than three or four times before a surface dive. More than this reduces the carbon dioxide level so much that your body may deplete oxygen to the point of hypoxia and unconsciousness before the carbon dioxide level in the blood rises to the level that tells you to breathe.

This is called "shallow water blackout" because it happens in shallow water to free divers. A surface diver who has excessively hyperventilated before a dive passes out when the oxygen available is no longer sufficient to maintain consciousness. Unfortunately, this event occurs before there is a build-up of carbon dioxide sufficient to stimulate the air hunger mentioned above.

The lesson to learn from shallow water blackout is that you should never hyperventilate when skin diving. A second lesson is that whenever you feel the need to breathe, head for the surface and satisfy that need. Never ignore the need for air.

Uncontrolled Hyperventilation

Hyperventilation is not always controlled. Sometimes simple anxiety and physical stress can cause it, whether the diver wants to hyperventilate or not. Anxiety or stress can make a person breathe quickly, which causes carbon dioxide to drop. Even unfamiliar equipment or a strange and unusual diving environment can cause hyperventilation.

Treating uncontrolled hyperventilation is easy because all you have to do is to stop doing anything that generates stress, and take control of your breathing. Consciously maintaining a slow, deep breathing pattern for a short time will help get the carbon dioxide level back to normal. It may be necessary to rebreathe your own air (using a paper bag) to bring the level of carbon dioxide back up to normal.

PANIC AND EXHAUSTION

Panic is defined as "unreasonable action usually caused by a blind, unreasoning fear." You lose control, you cannot think, and you therefore take incorrect actions. You focus on one particular task or action that may or may not have anything to do with escaping the problem. No matter how well you are trained or experienced, you are not immune to panic. The best way to prevent panic is to understand it and catch it early.

Fear is an ordinary, healthy response to danger. A fear of falling off a cliff is normal; stepping back from the edge of the cliff is a normal response. If the fear of falling causes you to freeze at the edge of the cliff, you have panicked and lost control. Panic is not a healthy response.

Avoiding panic, then, is largely a matter of controlling ordinary fear. If something goes wrong during a dive, you should recognize the normal fear for what it is and do what has to be done to correct the situation. Running out of air, difficulty with strong currents, excessive negative buoyancy from a full collecting bag, extreme cold, entanglement in kelp or a wreck, and equipment problems are all situations that have sensible and logical solutions. To solve any problem, however, you must be calm enough to think your way out of it. Panic is never a solution.

Recognizable signs of panic in either yourself or a buddy are a wide-eyed look, very rapid breathing, and undirected action. The breathing may look like hyperventilation but, when the diver is panicking, breathing is usually shallow, not deep. This, combined with uncontrolled action, leads to a build-up of carbon dioxide and a decrease in oxygen in the blood and tissues, which soon causes exhaustion. Exhaustion increases the panic and starts a vicious cycle which easily leads to disaster. Panic, in fact, is probably the leading cause of drowning and near drowning in sport diving. Drowning has been responsible for over one-half of all nonoccupational fatal diving accidents in the United States since 1970.

If, at any time during a dive, you feel anxious or are having difficulty in any way, *stop and think*. Relax and *breathe slowly and deeply until you have solved the problem and have regained complete control.*

Prevention is usually the best way to avoid problems that lead to anxiety while diving. Know your physical limitations and do not exceed them when diving. Do not wear poorly fitting or uncomfortable equipment because it adds stress to your diving. Keep your equipment maintained and in top working order. The *Advanced Manual* contains a more in-depth discussion of controlling diver stress and panic.

FIRST AID FOR DROWNING

Asphyxia is defined as the lack of oxygen in breathing air to the point where life is threatened. When the cause of asphyxia is water, it is referred to as drowning. Near drowning is the term applied to an individual who survives for a period of at least 24 hours after water-caused asphyxia.

In a drowning or near drowning, the victim will typically be unconscious and not breathing. Since the victim's heart may continue to beat for several minutes after breathing has stopped, artificial ventilation immediately is the most important element of first aid for a drowning.

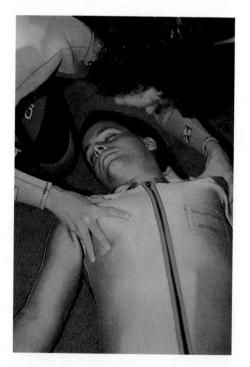

Fig. 7-4 *The first step is to determine whether or not the victim has simply fainted. Roll the victim to a face-up position on a firm surface such as the deck of a boat or pool or the firm sand on a beach. Gently shake the victim and shout into an ear, "Hey, are you OK?" If the victim has simply fainted, he or she will usually regain consciousness immediately or soon after lying down. If the victim does not respond or regain consciousness, ask bystanders to notify whatever emergency medical services are available to assist and then continue with the process of caring for the victim.*

Do not hesitate for any reason. The cells of the brain, heart, and lungs can suffer irreparable damage if deprived of oxygen for more than 4 to 6 minutes. It is important to begin artificial ventilation immediately.

CARDIOPULMONARY RESUSCITATION (CPR)

Artificial ventilation is done by mouth-to-mouth resuscitation and artificial circulation is done by external cardiac massage. Together, they are called cardiopulmonary resuscitation (CPR). The procedure is described below to acquaint you with how a victim is given CPR.

Though the material presented in Figs. 7-4 to 7-10 is quite thorough, you

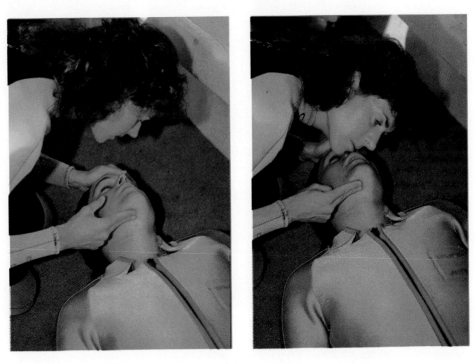

7-5   7-6

Fig. 7-5 *The second step is to open the victim's airway to help him or her breathe. Do this with the head-tilt, chin-lift method which puts your hand (the one closer to the victim's head) on the victim's forehead while two or three fingers of the other hand are placed under the victim's jaw as shown. By lifting with the fingers under the jaw and, at the same time, pressing gently on the victim's forehead, the head is rotated back to a hyperextended position. This lifts the tongue and keeps it from blocking the airway of the victim. Sometimes, opening the airway is enough to start victims breathing on their own.*

Fig. 7-6 *Step 3 is to put your ear very close to the victim's mouth and nose, while watching the victim's chest for the rise and fall of breathing for 3 to 5 seconds. Listen and feel for the noise and movement of air through the victim's mouth and nose.*

should obtain specialized training in CPR from the American Heart Association, the American National Red Cross, or the equivalent organization in your country if you are not being trained in the United States.

The purpose of CPR is to supply the victim's body with oxygen and, if necessary, establish and maintain the victim's circulation until normal breathing and heart beat are restored.

CPR is continued as shown in Figs. 7-4 to 7-10 until the victim begins to breathe spontaneously, the rescuer is too weak to continue or is relieved by some-

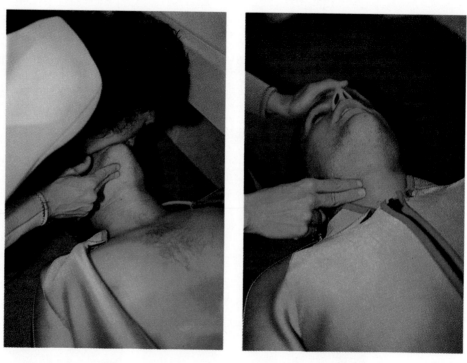

7-7   7-8

Fig. 7-7 *If the victim is not breathing, initiate mouth-to-mouth breathing by pinching the victim's nostrils closed with the hand you already have on the victim's forehead. Then cover the victim's mouth with your own and give two full ventilations, or rescue breaths. These breaths are slow, full ventilations taking 1 to 1½ seconds per breath. After each of these breaths, allow the victim to exhale.*

Fig. 7-8 *Immediately after the two rescue breaths, check the victim's pulse to learn if the heart is still beating. Do this by sliding two fingertips gently into the groove-like indentation between the trachea and the large muscle running down the side of the neck. There you will be able to feel the carotid pulse if the heart is still beating. If you feel a pulse, then the heart is still beating, and you need not perform chest compressions. However, if the victim is still not breathing then give rescue breaths at a rate of one breath every 5 seconds (12 breaths per minute). You should also recheck the pulse every few minutes to be certain the victim's heart is still beating.*

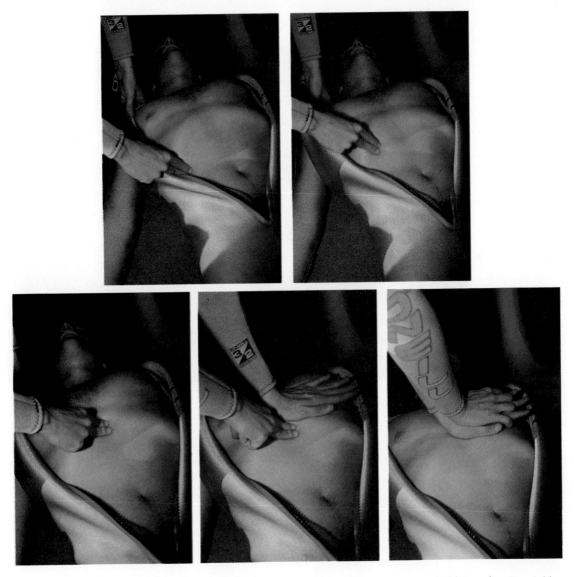

Fig. 7-9 If you do not feel a pulse, then the victim's heart is probably not beating. Initiate chest compressions along with mouth-to-mouth resuscitation. Expose the chest if it is not already bared. With two fingertips of your hand closest to the victim's feet, draw those fingertips along the lower border of the victim's rib cage until you come to the V-shaped base of the sternum (breastbone) in the midline of the body. Keep those two fingers where they are now resting (on the xiphoid process, the lowest segment of the sternum), and place the heel of your other hand, which is closest to the patient's head, on the sternum immediately next to the two fingers resting on the xiphoid process.

Now place the hand that is closest to the victim's feet on top of the hand already resting on the sternum. You may find it helps to interlock your fingers to avoid putting pressure on the ribs. Compress the sternum at a rate of 80 to 100 strokes per minute. Each stroke should compress the chest at least 1½ inches but not more than 2 inches.

After compressing the victim's chest for 15 strokes, ventilate the victim two more times as described in Fig. 7-7, then continue alternating 15 chest compressions with two ventilations. After four cycles of compressions and ventilations, recheck the pulse in the same manner as described in Fig. 7-8. If the pulse has returned, then stop chest compressions but continue mouth-to-mouth as needed. If there has been no return of pulse then ventilate the patient twice as in Fig. 7-7 and continue the chest compressions and mouth-to-mouth.

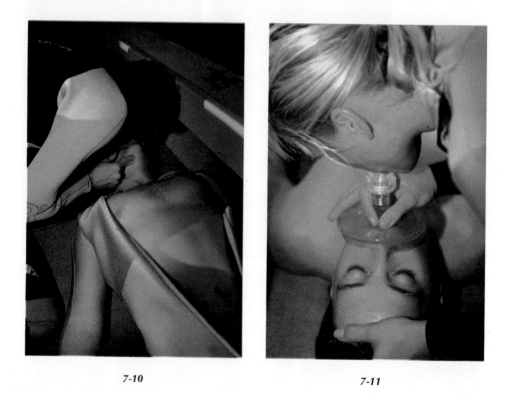

7-10   7-11

Fig. 7-10 *The rescuer gives the victim the two ventilations needed after every 15 compressions.*

Fig. 7-11 *Mouth-to-mask ventilation should be used when there is any concern about the risk of infection.*

one else who knows how to do cardiopulmonary resuscitation, or until the victim is placed in the hands of emergency medical services personnel.

If infection risk is a concern, then mouth-to-mouth can be done using a pocket mask device with a one-way valve as illustrated in Fig. 7-11. Except for the utilization of a mask, all other methods are the same as described above.

Mouth-to-mouth resuscitation can be started in the water as illustrated in Fig. 7-12. The mask may be carried in a BC pocket and utilized in resuscitative attempts. However, there is no universal agreement that such resuscitative efforts are useful. Perhaps it would be better to establish the airway for the victim, provide the two initial slow, full ventilations that might stimulate a return of spontaneous breathing, and then concentrate on moving the victim to the boat or shore for further resuscitative efforts. On the other hand, in the water the presence or absence of a pulse may be difficult to check (cold water, gloves, and so on) and if the victim is not breathing but does have heart activity, mouth-to-mask ventilation may be all that is required. Additionally, since pulses at the carotid artery are not generally palpable at very low blood pressures, there may still be circulation which

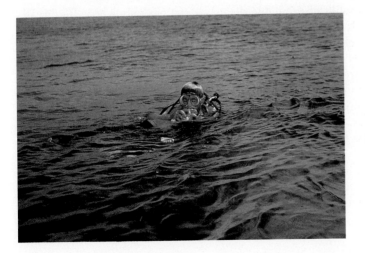

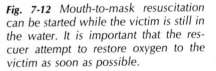
Fig. 7-12 *Mouth-to-mask resuscitation can be started while the victim is still in the water. It is important that the rescuer attempt to restore oxygen to the victim as soon as possible.*

simply cannot be felt. You should be guided by the rescue training adopted by the diving agency training you, since this is the standard against which a rescuer's performance will most likely be evaluated.

The material presented here only scratches the surface of rescue as it applies to scuba diving. A more comprehensive discussion of scuba rescue is presented in the *Advanced Manual* or will be a part of a rescue specialty course that you may pursue in the future.

CLEAN AIR

Sport divers should never breathe any gas underwater except clean, dry, filtered air. It must have only minimal levels of carbon monoxide, carbon dioxide, oil, vapor, and any other impurities that can cause short- and long-term health problems. (See "Air Purity Standards" in the Appendix.) Scuba tanks should never be filled with anything except ordinary air; other gases or gas mixtures should not be put in them.

From the time air is compressed by an air compressor until you inhale it from the regulator mouthpiece, there are a number of ways it can become contaminated. Here is a list of ways to prevent contamination:

1. Make sure the scuba air compressor air intake is located in an area free of gasoline engine exhaust fumes from an automobile, electric generator, boat, compressor engine, and the like. The fumes contain carbon monoxide gas that combines with the oxygen-carrying agent (hemoglobin) in red blood cells 200 times more effectively than oxygen. This means that carbon monoxide is carried in the blood and to the body's tissues in preference to oxygen, with the result that the cells are poisoned as well as being deprived of oxygen. Carbon monoxide poisoning, as it is called, can lead to unconsciousness and death.

2. Fill your scuba tanks at reputable diving air stations only where the breathing air leaving the compressor is filtered to remove any undesirable gases, water, oil, particles, and odor. The filtering process is designed to leave the air in a relatively pure state of being colorless, tasteless, odorless, and essentially moisture free to protect your body and your equipment from harm.

3. Before connecting your scuba tank to a filling hose, blow the valve clear of moisture and contaminants with tank air and do likewise with the filling hose using system air. This practice prevents moisture and contaminants from entering the scuba tank from air station compressor and storage tanks shown in Fig. 7-13.

4. Lubricate scuba regulators only with special breathing apparatus lubricants. Oil or grease used inside a regulator can find its way into the lungs and cause a type of pneumonia. Ordinary lubricating oils are not for scuba regulators.

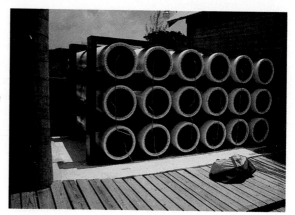

Fig. 7-13 *The bank of air storage cylinders at a modern diving facility.*

SUMMARY

The act of breathing and the process of respiration provide the cells of the body with the necessary oxygen to utilize their life-giving fuels to sustain life. In the absence of oxygen or in the presence of gases that are toxic, the body's machinery breaks down and stops working. That is why smart divers are so sensitive to and aware of the breathing process.

8 Descending and Ascending

- Effects of Pressure Change
- Boyle's Law
- Squeezes
- Air Embolism
- Ascent Procedures

OBJECTIVES

At the conclusion of Chapter 8, you will be able to:

1. State the weight in psi that the atmosphere exerts on the earth's surface.

2. State the number of feet of salt water and the number of feet of fresh water necessary to exert 1 atmosphere.

3. Explain the difference between absolute pressure and gauge pressure.

4. State the fractional volume of a closed container filled with air when it is taken from the surface to a depth of 33 feet in salt water.

5. Explain how the phenomenon referred to in point 4 will affect your middle ear when you dive and what you can do while descending to prevent this from injuring you.

6. State what will happen to a container which is filled with air and sealed at a depth of 33 fsw and then brought to the surface.

7. Name two conditions that can result from the above.

8. Name one thing that you must never do while scuba diving that might cause the conditions referred to in point 7.

9. State the common cause of air embolism when using scuba.

10. State, from memory, the emergency phone number for the Divers Alert Network.

KEY TERMS

Atmosphere	Absolute pressure	Gauge pressure
Ambient pressure	Ear squeeze	Sinus squeeze
Air embolism	Pneumothorax	DAN

EFFECTS OF PRESSURE CHANGE

Even though people live in a pressurized environment, pressure is rarely noticed until it changes. Many people become aware of changes in pressure while driving up or down steep hills, and even more feel changes in cabin pressure aboard airplanes in flight. The change we feel is usually in our ears.

Divers feel the changes in both air and water pressure almost as soon as they put their heads underwater. These changes have important effects. This chapter tells you how water pressure and air pressure affect each other and your body, so you can handle them more confidently and effectively.

Air Pressure and Water Pressure

To say that air and water exert pressure is to say that they exert a force on an area. In the United States, pressure is usually measured in pounds per square inch, which is abbreviated "psi." The metric measurement most frequently used in the same context is kilograms per square centimeter.

At sea level, ordinary air pressure exerts a force of 14.7 psi. In other words, the column of air extending as high as the earth's atmospheric envelope, approximately 60 miles, "presses" toward the earth with a force of 14.7 pounds on a 1 × 1 inch square area, as shown in Fig. 8-1. This air pressure of 14.7 psi is also called 1 atmosphere of pressure, at sea level.

Salt water, because it is so much heavier than air, exerts 1 atmosphere of pressure with a 1 × 1 inch column only 33 feet high, as shown in Fig. 8-2. Because fresh water is slightly less dense, it requires a 1 × 1 inch column 34 feet high to exert the same pressure of 1 atmosphere (14.7 psi). Thus, a 60-mile column of air, a 34-foot column of fresh water, and a 33-foot column of salt water all exert the same pressure—1 atmosphere at sea level.

The total amount of pressure exerted on a diver depends on how much air and water are pressing down at any given time, as shown in Fig. 8-3. At an altitude of 18,000 feet, for example, there is only one-half the amount of air pressure that there is at sea level, i.e., 7.35 psi, or one-half atmosphere. Diving in high altitude lakes, above 3,000 feet, requires special techniques not used at sea level.

At an underwater depth of 66 feet in sea water, the total pressure is exerted by 1 atmosphere of air stacked on 2 atmospheres of water pressure. Together, the water and air pressures exert a total of 3 atmospheres of absolute pressure (44.1 psi). This is called absolute pressure because it refers to a measurement of the total pressure exerted. At 33 feet depth in sea water, for example, the absolute pressure would be 2 atmospheres (1 atmosphere of water and 1 atmosphere of air), or 29.4 psi absolute (14.7 psi of water and 14.7 psi of air).

Ambient pressure is another term used to express the total pressure surrounding a diver. It is usually expressed in absolute pressure or psia. At sea level, for example, the ambient pressure is 14.7 psia. At 33 feet under sea water, the ambient pressure surrounding a diver is 29.4 psia.

Gauge pressure differs from ambient and absolute by 14.7 psi because it refers to the pressure indicated by a gauge which is calibrated to show zero pressure on the surface of the earth. The zero mark on a pressure gauge, therefore, represents air pressure at normal atmospheric pressure. On the pressure gauge, then, 500 psi really means 500 psi above atmospheric air pressure.

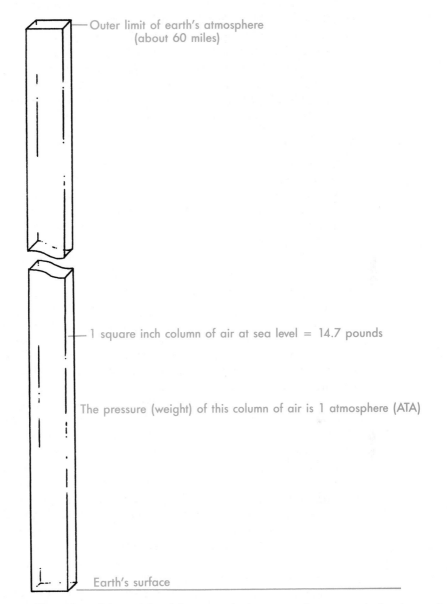

Fig. 8-1 *Illustration of the weight of the atmospheric pressure in a square-inch column of air which is stated as 1 atmosphere of pressure.*

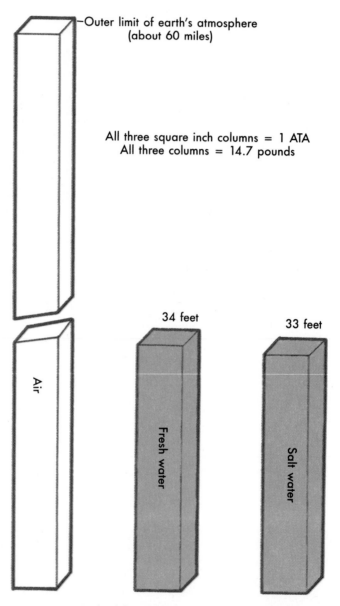

Outer limit of earth's atmosphere
(about 60 miles)

All three square inch columns = 1 ATA
All three columns = 14.7 pounds

Air

34 feet

33 feet

Fresh water

Salt water

Fig. 8-2 Each of these columns weighs 14.7 pounds.

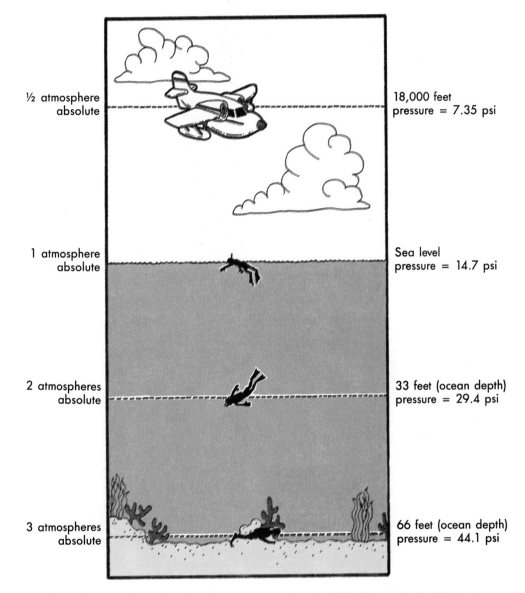

½ atmosphere absolute — 18,000 feet pressure = 7.35 psi

1 atmosphere absolute — Sea level pressure = 14.7 psi

2 atmospheres absolute — 33 feet (ocean depth) pressure = 29.4 psi

3 atmospheres absolute — 66 feet (ocean depth) pressure = 44.1 psi

Fig. 8-3 *A comparison of various pressures at an altitude of 18,000 to a depth of 66 feet in sea water.*

Increasing Pressure

When you descend below the surface, in sea water, pressure increases by 1 atmosphere every 33 feet. One effect of this increasing pressure can be easily demonstrated.

Take, for example, a standard, plastic milk jug, as shown in Figs. 8-4 through 8-6. If you fill the jug with air, seal it, then take it under the water, the effect of pressure becomes quite evident. The jug is crushed more and more the further you descend.

The reason that a water-filled container would not collapse in the same manner is that water is virtually incompressible. You cannot "squeeze" it or force it into a smaller space. Pressure against a water-filled container is transmitted to and through the water inside the container. No matter how great the pressure, the water stays the same size.

Air, or any gas for that matter, is compressible. Pressure squeezes it into a much smaller volume. As is evident from Fig. 8-6 above, the force of 3 atmospheres absolute is enough to squeeze the air into a space that is one-third the size of the original container. The air in the container is squeezed until the air pressure inside equals the surrounding water pressure outside, then the squeezing action stops. This squeezing causes the volume of the gas to be compressed into a smaller space thereby putting the gas molecules closer together. This increases the density of the gas; the gas is packed into a smaller space.

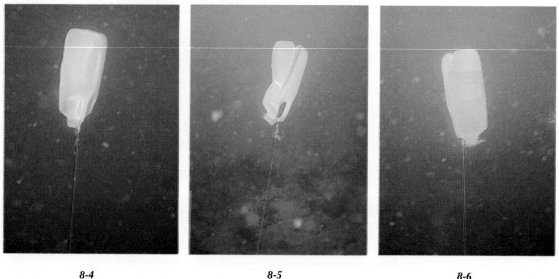

8-4   8-5   8-6

Fig. 8-4 This sealed jug has been taken to 33 feet (2 ATA), where it has been crushed to half its original volume.

Fig. 8-5 At 66 feet (3 ATA), the jug is crushed to a third of its original volume.

Fig. 8-6 An open jug taken to 33 feet (2 ATA) has the air inside compressed to half its original volume with water displacing the compressed air.

BOYLE'S LAW

In 1610, Robert Boyle, a British physicist and chemist, noticed the pressure effect on containers of air and other gases. He found the same effect every time gas was compressed and developed a mathematical formula to express this relationship. It is now known as "Boyle's Law."

The law states that if the temperature stays the same, the volume of a gas gets smaller in the same proportion that the surrounding pressure increases. (See the section on gas laws in the Appendix.)

Boyle's Law is illustrated in Figs. 8-7 through 8-9. A container filled with air is turned upside down so water can enter it freely and compress the air as water pressure increases. The reason the container does not completely fill with water immediately is that the compressed air within the container becomes denser and exerts a pressure against the water equal to the ambient pressure. At 33 feet (2 ATA, 29.4 psia), the volume of air is cut in half because the water pressure has doubled to force water to fill half of the container (doubling the density of the air). At 66 feet (3 ATA, 44.1 psia), the air is compressed to one-third its original volume. When you return the container to the surface, the air expands to its original volume.

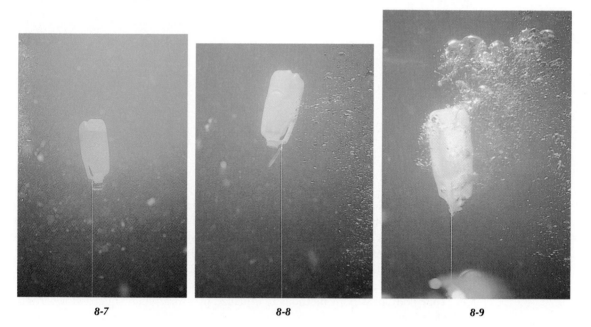

8-7   8-8   8-9

Fig. 8-7 *At 66 feet (3 ATA), the air is now compressed to a third of its original volume.*

Fig. 8-8 *This jug was filled with compressed air at 66 feet (3 ATA) and sealed at that depth. As ascent begins, the jug begins to stretch as the volume of the air expands with ascent.*

Fig. 8-9 *At approximately 33 feet (2 ATA), the volume of the air is 1.5 times as great as it was at 66 feet and the jug fails structurally, with the air escaping from the ruptured jug into the surrounding water.*

Boyle's Law is significant for the diver in several ways. Most of your body can be thought of as a large liquid-filled "body balloon." Like a water-filled container, nothing significant happens to the water-filled portion of your body during descent. Increasing pressure is simply transmitted into and through blood, bone, and solid tissue without damaging anything. No one knows exactly how much pressure the human body can withstand, but in experimental diving settings, humans have survived exposures greater than 1,900 feet. This is well beyond sport diving depth.

Boyle's Law, however, does affect the air spaces of your body. There are air-filled spaces in the ears, sinuses, lungs and airways, and stomach and intestines, as shown in Fig. 8-10. All of these spaces tend to respond to pressure in the same way the air-filled container did—they are all subject to "squeezes."

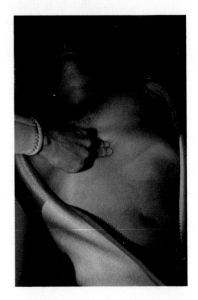

Fig. 8-10 *Air spaces within the diver's body including the ears, sinuses, lungs, airways, stomach, and intestines.*

SQUEEZES

Boyle's Law implies that air spaces will tend to equalize with the surrounding ambient pressure. This equalization can take place in two ways: (1) the space itself can become smaller or (2) more air can be put into the space to increase the pressure to that of ambient. At 33 feet, for example, the air-filled container is either squeezed to one-half its initial volume or it would have to contain twice the air in order to equalize with the ambient water pressure, since the air is two times as dense at 33 feet. Your body uses both methods to equalize pressure when squeezed according to Boyle's Law.

Ear Squeeze

The middle ear is an air space connected to the back of your throat by the eustachian tube, which is usually short. (Note Fig. 8-11.) An ear squeeze occurs when increasing water pressure pushes against the eardrum without being equalized. In extreme cases, the pressure can break the eardrum. Sometimes a rupture can even

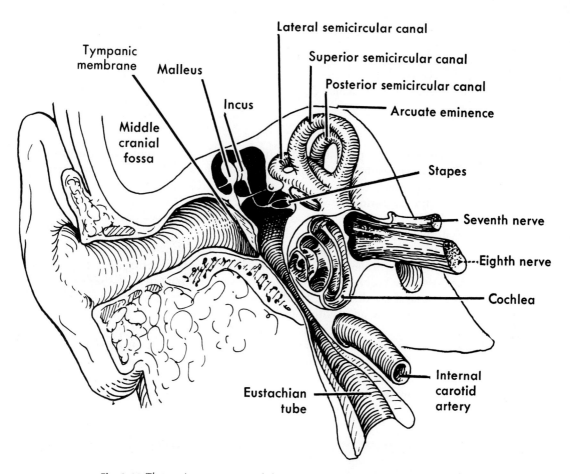

Fig. 8-11 *The major structures of the ear. (Modified from DeWeese DD and Saunders WH: Textbook of otolaryngology, ed 3, St. Louis, 1968, The CV Mosby Co.)*

occur in the inner ear. An inner ear rupture may cause permanent deafness.

Putting more air into the middle ear space is the way to equalize pressure. Yawning or swallowing sometimes opens the eustachian tube enough to allow air to enter the middle ear to equalize pressure. Usually, it is necessary to close your nose and mouth, and gently blow against your closed nose. This pushes equalizing air up your eustachian tubes, into the middle ear. (See Chapter 1.) You can try that on land, too. You will know you have sent air to your middle ear when your ears suddenly feel full and your hearing changes. Yawning or swallowing should relieve the full feeling in your ears and your hearing back to normal.

On a dive, it is prudent to anticipate ear squeeze. Begin by flexing your eustachian tubes by equalizing at the surface before you even descend. As you descend, equalize once for every foot you go down or with every exhalation. Do not wait for discomfort to start or pain to tell you to equalize. Waiting to equalize till one feels a pressure change may be too late for people with ear problems. Follow the rule "equalize early and often."

Colds, allergic reactions, infections, eating mucus-producing foods such as dairy products, and other factors can block the eustachian tubes and make it impossible to equalize. If you cannot equalize, do not dive. The injury you prevent is your own.

Sinus Squeeze

Another set of air spaces is located in the nasal areas around the eyes, as shown in Fig. 8-12. These air spaces, called sinuses, are surrounded by bone and lined with a membrane connected to the nasal cavity. Like the middle ear, they must be filled with extra gas during descent to prevent a painful sinus squeeze.

Usually they will equalize as you descend, because air passes freely from your nasal cavity into the sinuses. Colds, allergies, and infections, however, sometimes swell the nose and sinus membranes to prevent that air passage.

In this case, some divers use decongestants, nose drops, sprays, or pills to open the passages. Problems can result, however, from the use of drugs underwater. One is that if the decongestant effect wears off too soon, your sinuses may trap air inside on the way up. Another is drowsiness caused in some people when they use decongestants containing antihistamines. To avoid either of these problems, it is best to postpone your dive until you can equalize without medications.

If you must use any medication for diving, consult a physician familiar with diving medicine first, to discover any adverse effects the medication may have on your diving. Some medicines act differently in the body when under pressure. If you

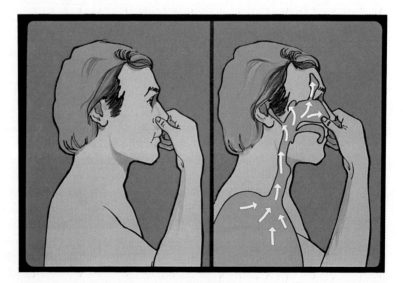

Fig. 8-12 The paranasal sinuses are interconnected with the nasal cavity and are equalized during the descent in much the same manner as the ears.

must dive using some sort of sinus medication, be certain that the physician can assure you that the medication's effect lasts long enough to take you well beyond the anticipated duration of your dive.

Lung Squeeze

Compared to the middle ear and sinus cavities, the lungs are flexible, so they tend to equalize by changing volume instead of adding air. When you descend on a breath-hold dive, the increasing water pressure ordinarily reduces the size of the lungs and compresses the air inside until it is automatically equalized with ambient pressure.

Breath-hold divers have gone below 300 feet with no damage to their lungs. Constant breathing with scuba equipment continuously replenishes the lungs with adequate air which, in turn, eliminates the possibility of lung squeeze.

Stomach and Intestine Squeezes

Digesting food often produces gas bubbles or pockets in the stomach and intestines, which are "squeezed" harmlessly during descent because they are surrounded by flexible tissue. If gas continues to form at depth, however, it will expand on your return to the surface. This can be painful and calls for a slow ascent to let the bubbles or pockets move away from sensitive areas. To prevent this kind of squeeze, stay away from gas-producing foods before diving.

Equipment Squeezes

Artificial air spaces next to the body can cause squeezes the same way internal air spaces can. The mask squeeze, for example, can damage tissues around and in the eyes.

A preoccupied diver might not notice the pain caused by mask squeeze until the damage has been done. A mask squeeze is easily prevented by simply exhaling a bit through your nose into the mask to equalize pressure within the mask during descent. (See Chapter 1.) Not equalizing causes facial and eye tissues to fill the space of the compressed air, to conform to Boyle's Law. The result is facial bruising and ruptured small blood vessels in the face and the eyes as the tissues are squeezed.

Never wear goggles or earplugs while scuba diving. The air spaces created by these devices *cannot be equalized,* so the eye tissues or eardrums will be damaged by the increased pressure change as stated in Boyle's Law. Air can also be trapped in the outer ear by a tightly fitting exposure suit hood. To prevent hood squeeze, pull the hood away from the head to let some water pressure in. Some divers have cut small holes in their hoods next to the ears.

Another common equipment squeeze is that associated with a dry suit. The dry suit keeps a layer of air next to the diver's body. Upon descent, this air space is compressed, thereby requiring more air to prevent the suit from getting too snug. If this air is not added, the suit may be crushed over a fold of skin to cause a suit-squeeze welt. If you are planning to buy or use a dry suit, seek proper instruction from a qualified instructor or dive products retailer. Always follow the manufacturer's instructions on care and maintenance.

Tooth Squeeze

Tooth squeeze, though extremely rare, in theory is caused by a small pocket of trapped gas in a decayed tooth or underneath a cracked filling. If this air bubble is not equalized, increasing pressure squeezes the soft pulp of the tooth into the space to create pain, or may result in damage to dental work if the bubble expands significantly. It is also possible that pain apparently originating in the teeth during diving may be a result of referred pain from barotrauma to the sinuses or poor equalization of the sinuses during ascent or descent.

VERTIGO

Vertigo can be caused by a pressure imbalance in the ears. It may also follow an eardrum rupture as cold water enters the middle ear. Eardrum rupture is preceded by pain, which may actually diminish when the rupture occurs. Dizziness, disorientation, and nausea are some of the symptoms of vertigo. These stop, in cases of eardrum rupture, when the water which entered the ear upon rupture, warms up. During vertigo, you should breathe normally and hang onto something stationary until the disorienting feelings pass. If pain was present just before the onset of the vertigo and is now gone, you should terminate your dive and see a doctor to determine if eardrum injury has occurred.

DECREASING PRESSURE

During ascent, when pressure decreases, air naturally expands according to Boyle's Law. Suppose we fill a container with compressed air at 66 feet (3 ATA, 44.1 psi) and bring it up. Since air at this depth is compressed to only one-third its sea level volume, the container holds 1½ gallons of sea level air. As the container is brought up, the air expands.

The container is sealed at 66 feet after being filled with compressed air. As it ascends, it begins to bulge, stretch, and leak and finally bursts, allowing the expanding air to escape.

The ears, sinuses, mask, and lungs usually let the expanding air escape into the surrounding environment without the need for any equalizing effort. But if the air spaces are closed off like the sealed container, a "reverse" squeeze takes place and surrounding tissues may be damaged. Always breathe continuously and naturally during ascent. Even during "out of air" ascents you must keep the airway open by exhaling continuously all the way to the surface. This prevents overexpansion injury to the lungs.

AIR EMBOLISM

If you should hold your breath on a scuba ascent, your lungs become like the sealed container and can overexpand and burst. Therefore, continuing to breathe at all times while scuba diving will enable you to prevent the situation described below.

When you hold your breath, structures within your throat close off the lungs to the outside world. During a scuba diving ascent, holding your breath can cause tearing or rupturing of your lungs because of the expanding air they contain.

If the air escapes from the alveoli directly into the small vessels surrounding the alveoli, it can then travel through the pulmonary veins, into the heart. From the heart, air can then travel up the carotid arteries in the neck and eventually may find its way into the small arteries and capillaries of the brain. Embolism comes from the word embolus, which means "plug." If these bubbles are circulating during ascent, they follow Boyle's Law and continue to expand as pressure decreases. The air bubble or bubbles get stuck in a small artery or capillary and will form a plug, which cuts off blood supply to the part of the brain supplied by the blocked vessel as illustrated in Fig. 8-13. This can be extremely serious and can lead to unconsciousness and death.

AIR BUBBLES MOVE FROM LUNGS TO HEART, TO BRAIN

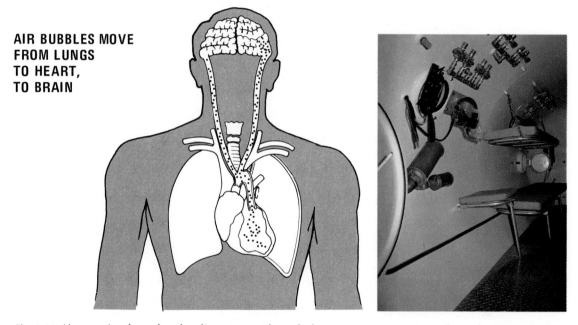

Fig. 8-13 Air escaping from the alveoli can move through the heart to the brain and plug vessels supplying parts of the brain.

Fig. 8-14 Immediate recompression in a chamber is the treatment for air embolism.

The only effective treatment for air embolism is *immediate* recompression in a chamber, as shown in Fig. 8-14. Inside the chamber, the pressure is increased very quickly to the equivalent of 165 feet of sea water to reduce the diameter of the air bubbles so they will not plug the blood vessels or so that blood flow may be restored if it has already been stopped. Then the pressure is gradually reduced and the diver is decreased to ambient pressure.

First Aid for Air Embolism

Since air embolism is life-threatening, let us discuss the symptoms and first aid for this emergency.

Symptoms of air embolism usually occur in a matter of seconds after the diver surfaces and may even occur during ascent. The diver may experience weakness, dizziness, paralysis, changes in vision, chest pain, frothy pink blood in the mouth, seizures, and cessation of breathing and may eventually lose consciousness.

Whenever there is the slightest chance that a diver could have experienced an air embolism, take the following first aid measures and get the injured diver to a recompression chamber as soon as possible. Do not try to recompress the victim in the water because the debilitating symptoms of air embolism are not compatible with being underwater.

1. Lay the victim flat on the back on a firm surface and do a primary survey (ABCs).
2. Perform cardiopulmonary resuscitation as needed.
3. Administer 100 percent oxygen to the breathing victim or during CPR. Ideally this should be done utilizing the manually triggered, positive pressure, demand valve device, but only if you have been trained in its use.
4. Treat the patient for shock.
5. Immediately transport the victim to the nearest facility with a recompression chamber. If you are unsure where to go, contact the Divers Alert Network (DAN) at 919-684-8111. Physicians there will be able to guide you and give other treatment recommendations as appropriate.

The above procedure for management of a diving accident is dealt with in much greater detail in the *Advanced Manual*.

OTHER OVERPRESSURE INJURIES

Another way that air may escape from overexpanding lungs is for a tear to occur in the respiratory tree other than the alveoli, resulting in air passing into the mediastinum—the space in the middle of the chest cavity where the trachea, heart, and great vessels lie. Air in the mediastinum causes mediastinal emphysema, a problem that includes chest pain, breathing difficulties, and faintness because of air pressure against the heart; however, this is rarely a life-threatening problem.

A situation in which air is forced under the pericardium—the tissue surrounding the heart—also results in chest pain, breathing difficulties, and faintness due to pressure directly on the heart similar to pneumomediastinum, but this condition, called pneumopericardium, can cause life-threatening heart damage.

From the mediastinal area, air bubbles can travel up and under the skin in the neck, upper chest region, and face. This condition, called subcutaneous emphysema, may cause breathing difficulties, swelling, and even changes in the voice. When you press on the skin in the areas affected, it will feel much like pressing on bubble-wrap, the sheet material sometimes used to ship fragile objects.

If the lung tissues rupture and escaping air gets into the space between the lungs and chest wall, the condition is known as pneumothorax. The expanding air may not only collapse the lung in the part of the chest where the air is escaping, but the air might expand to the point where it pushes against the heart and affects circulation. The most common symptoms of this condition are chest pain and breathing difficulties.

For any of these conditions, the appropriate treatment is medical attention.

PREVENTION

In all diving accidents, prevention is much more effective than a cure. Any condition that could possibly interfere with air escaping easily from the lungs should be carefully evaluated before diving. Conditions such as pneumonia, asthma, lung scars, and even smoking can block the free flow of air out of alveoli and should be evaluated in a physical examination performed by a physician familiar with diving medicine. Your first physical should include a chest x-ray, especially if you are a smoker or have a family history of asthma or other associated lung diseases, and subsequent examinations should be done periodically to note changes. An RSTC (Recreational Scuba Training Council) medical form may be used as a guide for a physician not familiar with diving physiology.

Other prevention takes place in the water because the most common cause of air embolism is breath holding while on scuba. It is entirely natural for an air-breathing creature to hold its breath underwater. In an emergency or panic situation, holding your breath is a powerfully strong instinct. It is important to fight this natural tendency whenever you scuba dive. *Never hold your breath while scuba diving.* Always breathe naturally with the regulator in your mouth. If the regulator is out of your mouth; be sure to *exhale* continuously.

As a matter of interest in preventing air embolism, remember that the greatest change in relative pressure occurs in shallow water. There is a 100 percent increase in pressure in the first 33 feet. In the next 33 feet, from 33 to 66 feet, pressure increases an additional 50 percent, or half the pressure increase in the first 33 feet. The deeper you go, the smaller the relative change in pressure. The danger of embolism, then, is greater in shallow water where the most dramatic changes in pressure exist. Embolism has occurred in water as shallow as 4 feet.

Ascent Procedures

In addition to proper breathing, proper ascent procedures will help you to avoid air embolism (Fig. 8-15). Every routine ascent should follow these steps:

1. Confirm with your buddy that it is time to surface.
2. Check the time and prepare to monitor your depth gauge or computer as you ascend.
3. With neutral or slightly positive buoyancy, face your buddy and look up for a clear route to the surface.
4. Raise your inflator hose above your head and put your thumb on the deflator button in preparation to vent air from your BC.
5. Kick your fins to begin your ascent and start your ascent. Rates of ascent vary depending upon the table being utilized. Some computers employ a table recommending a maximum rate of ascent of 20 feet per minute from depths of 60 feet or less. The U.S. Navy and DCIEM tables utilize an ascent rate of 60 feet per minute. Other tables use ascent rates of 30 feet per minute from 50 feet to the surface while still others recommend a uniform ascent rate of 40 feet per minute (12 meters per minute) *or less.* Keep the inflator hose raised and continue to look toward the surface for obstructions while monitoring your rate of ascent.

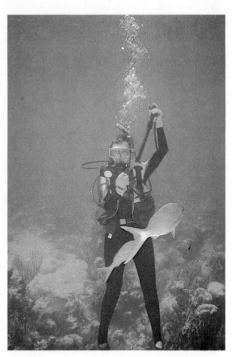

Fig. 8-15 *This diver is using proper ascent techniques by monitoring ascent rate, having the inflator hose extended, and looking toward the surface during the ascent for any possible obstruction.*

6. Breathe regularly and continuously while ascending and let expanding air vent from your BC to maintain your slow rate of ascent.
7. On all dives it is a good idea to make a safety stop at 15 feet for 2 minutes. On dives to depths greater than 40 feet, make a neutrally buoyant safety stop of not less than 3 minutes at 15 feet, then slowly continue to the surface.
8. If you ascend without your buddy, follow exactly the same procedures as above but turn 360 degrees during your ascent to see that you have a clear path to the surface.

When you reach the surface but before taking the regulator out of your mouth, inflate your BC to establish positive buoyancy. Depending upon water conditions, you may wish to switch from your regulator to snorkel, but in extremely rough water conditions it may be best to keep your regulator in place.

Signal the boat or beach with the OK sign if everything is under control and continue to be ready to provide your buddy with any necessary assistance. This is especially important at the end of a dive when you are both tired.

Emergency Ascents

Emergency ascents made when you are out of air are somewhat different. You can ascend by yourself or with the help of your buddy. Here are the various options you have to choose from in order of preference:

1. Sharing your buddy's air by the use of an octopus or alternate air source as discussed in Chapter 3

2. Sharing your buddy's air by buddy breathing (see Chapter 3)
3. Emergency swimming ascent alone
4. Emergency buoyant ascent alone

Though emergency ascents will take you back to the surface, *not running out of air* along with a normal ascent is the best of all. Second best would be having a totally independent, alternate air source as part of your equipment.

Emergency Swimming Ascent. An emergency swimming ascent (ESA) is basically swimming to the surface on one breath, the last one you took when you realized you were out of air. An ESA depends primarily on kicking to get you to the surface.

You begin the emergency swimming ascent with a push off the bottom or with several strong kicks upward. *Keep the regulator in your mouth, look up, and alternate trying to breathe in from your regulator as you ascend while exhaling gently to avoid lung overexpansion.*

As you ascend, the reduction in ambient pressure allows the second stage of the regulator to deliver air from an apparently empty tank. A scuba tank at 99 feet of sea water has only one fourth of its working volume of air available. As a result, you can probably get a breath or two on your way up. Try to inhale as you ascend, but be careful to exhale at all other times to prevent air embolism.

Never hold your breath during any normal or emergency ascent but do not exhale all the air from your lungs, either. The objective is to keep your lungs at a normal volume. You should try to breathe in and out as you ascend.

Keep one hand on the quick-release buckle of your weight belt and be ready to use it to change your ascent into an emergency buoyant ascent.

Emergency Buoyant Ascent. An EBA is the same as an ESA except that you add buoyancy to help you to get to the surface quicker.

An EBA starts when you ditch your weight belt as described above (see Fig. 8-1), inflate your buoyancy compensator, or both. It is used if you have any doubts that you can reach the surface in time by ESA or buddy breathing ascent. The weight-dropping EBA does not allow you to control your rate of ascent as easily as ascents where you keep your weight belt. Loss of control in this manner increases the possibility of air embolism, lung overexpansion injuries, and decompression sickness.

Because of your increased speed during ascent, you should definitely exhale more rapidly and look up at the surface to avoid obstacles. Releasing air from your buoyancy compensator will help slow your ascent and keep the rate of ascent more controlled.

When you are about 20 feet from the surface, spread your arms out, your shoulders back, arch your back, and put your fins parallel to the surface. This "flares" your body and creates a lot of drag to slow your ascent. Flaring reduces your chances for injury as you approach the surface and come through that part of the water column with the greatest relative pressure decrease (Fig. 8-17). An EBA is *only* used if you have any doubt that you can reach the surface in time after considering buddy breathing and an emergency swimming ascent.

Selecting an Emergency Ascent. Since the best emergency ascent varies with the situation, a diver must practice and master each in order to have all ready for use in an emergency. Each of the basic ascent methods has its own advantages and disadvantages.

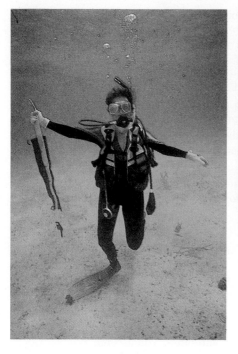

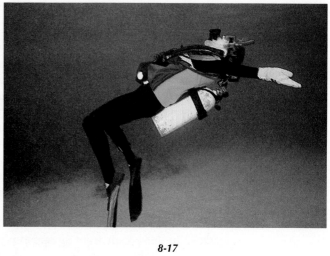

8-17

8-16

Fig. 8-16 *When the need to ditch the weight belt is made or if in the emergency swimming ascent you elect to hold the weight belt in your hand, make sure the belt is held away from your body so that it is clear of any possible entanglement with your equipment.*

Fig. 8-17 *During an emergency buoyant ascent the diver flares as the surface is approached to slow the rate of ascent.*

The primary advantages of the emergency swimming ascent are that it is fast, simple, and independent of your buddy. Its disadvantage is that it exposes you to lung overexpansion injuries.

The emergency buoyant ascent almost guarantees that you will arrive at the surface and stay there. The primary disadvantage to this method is that you ascend more rapidly than normal and with less control, thereby increasing the danger of collision, air embolism, and decompression sickness.

An emergency octopus ascent and emergency buddy breathing ascent both have the obvious advantage of supplying you with air throughout the emergency ascent. The octopus ascent is better since neither of you is deprived of an air supply at any time during the ascent, while buddy breathing with a single regulator may become frustrating and difficult, especially if the needer is in great stress and the buddy pair is not well trained. Buddy breathing is a skill that requires regular practice to maintain, without which it may become more hazardous than helpful in an emergency.

For out-of-air emergencies in caves or wrecks and under kelp or ice, the lack of direct access to the surface forces you to use buddy breathing with or without an octopus to survive. Cave, wreck, and ice diving are all specialized forms of diving that require extra training well beyond the scope of basic scuba instruction. In all three types of diving, the concept of redundancy is stressed so that in an emergency you have spare working equipment and in that regard are relatively self-sufficient. *Do not* attempt any of these forms of diving without intense specialized training from an authorized instructor.

SUMMARY

An out-of-air emergency should not occur except under catastrophic failure of the regulator, which is extremely rare.

Advances in emergency ascent procedures, buoyancy compensation equipment, and accident research and reporting have done much to increase diving safety. Day-to-day safety continues to depend mainly on good training and repeated practice.

Do not be satisfied with just becoming fairly familiar with emergency ascents. *Overlearn* a single reliable out-of-air technique that is best suited for your diving and learn the skill steps until they become second nature.

9 Depth and Time Limits

- Sport Diving Limits
- Nitrogen Narcosis
- Oxygen Tolerance
- Partial Pressures
- Decompression Sickness
- Altitude Diving
- Flying and Diving

OBJECTIVES

At the conclusion of Chapter 9, you will be able to:

1. Name the nitrogen problem that causes divers to act illogically or unsafely when at depths below 100 feet.
2. Name at least two symptoms of nitrogen narcosis.
3. Name the gas that is essential for life at sea level but can become toxic under extreme pressures.
4. Name the normally inert gas that, when it comes out of solution, results in decompression sickness.
5. Define bottom time.
6. Explain why diving at a high altitude may increase the risk of decompression sickness.
7. State how long a diver should wait after his or her last dive before flying.
8. Describe one of the reasons recompression is used to treat decompression sickness.
9. Explain why pure oxygen should be breathed by the diver suffering from decompression sickness.
10. State the maximum altitude at which diving is recommended using the U.S. Navy tables.

KEY TERMS

Oxygen toxicity	Caisson disease	Chokes
Paul Bert	Bends	Haldane
No-decompression limits	Ascent rates	Bottom time

Effects of Diving Too Deep and Too Long

The direct effects of increased pressure on the air spaces inside and outside the diver's body are obvious. Spaces become bigger and smaller almost immediately, and you can either see or feel the changes while they occur. There are, however, less obvious changes.

Pressure also affects gases and gas mixtures in the body in definite but invisible ways. These effects put limits on the mind and body. Even though you may not see these changes easily, they are paramount in planning and conducting safe dives.

Fortunately, the direct and indirect effects of breathing compressed air under water are measurable and generally predictable. Because they are generally predictable, certain depth and time limits can be set for sport divers. Staying within these limits is a nearly sure way to reduce any problems resulting from effects of pressure. The key to staying within the limits is to monitor your depth and time indicators, especially in areas of extremely clear water, where the bottom, 130 feet below, is clearly visible from the surface and "seems" to be within easy reach.

It is suggested that sport divers limit their diving to depths of less than 100 feet. Deeper diving, to be safe, requires more extensive training and sophisticated equipment than a normal certified sport diver has.

Though a 100-foot limit may sound restrictive, it really is not, especially if you are like most sport divers, who usually dive in waters shallower than 30 feet. They enjoy their dives in the warmer water, and more profuse marine life is usually found closer to the surface.

NITROGEN NARCOSIS

Ordinarily, nitrogen and other inert gases are inactive, that is, they are not consumed or used by the body. At depth, however, the increased pressure of nitrogen makes it a narcotic. A narcotic alters your ability to think and perceive. Even at depths only slightly greater than 100 feet, nitrogen narcosis has caused divers to take illogical and unsafe actions because of being "narked."

Symptoms and Prevention

The narcotic effects of nitrogen are easily measurable at even 60 feet of sea water (Fig. 9-1). Nitrogen narcosis, like alcohol intoxication, is dose related and varies from individual to individual. For many years, the diving community has explained this phenomenon using "Martini's Law"—diving to 50 feet is equivalent to drinking one dry martini; diving to 100 feet equals two dry martinis; and so on. Beyond 100 feet, nitrogen narcosis can affect your ability to think and make judgments; at 150 feet, you may become somewhat dizzy. Between 200 and 250 feet, you may become unable to communicate or perform simple motor or mental tasks, and below 250 feet, the average diver becomes a safety menace to himself or herself and others.

Several factors change your tolerance and resistance to nitrogen narcosis. Alcohol, a hangover, fatigue, excess carbon dioxide, inexperience, and anxiety tend to increase the narcotic effects. Different divers are affected by nitrogen narcosis in

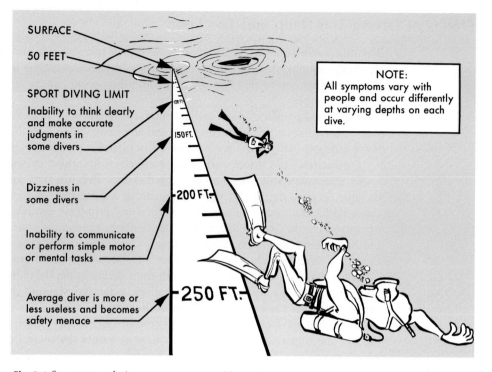

Fig. 9-1 *Symptoms of nitrogen narcosis and how they vary at depth.*

different ways. Any one diver may experience different symptoms on different dives and at different depths. Regardless of the diver or the symptoms, simply returning to shallower depths is the easiest way to both prevent and treat nitrogen narcosis.

OXYGEN TOLERANCE

The other main gas in a diver's air is oxygen, which the diver needs for survival. An excess of oxygen, however, is just as bad as too little. If you breathe an excess of oxygen for an extended period of time, it can injure lung tissues. At higher pressures, oxygen can adversely affect the central nervous system.

PARTIAL PRESSURES

How much oxygen is too much? This depends on two things: its pressure, and the exposure time.

Ordinarily, we breathe a mixture of 78 percent nitrogen and 21 percent oxygen at atmospheric pressure (14.7 psi). The oxygen in the mixture is 21 percent of 14.7 psi or 3.09 psi according to Dalton's Law, which states that the total pressure of a gas mixture equals the sum of the partial pressures that make up that mixture. The

3.09 psi is the partial pressure of oxygen, while the sea level partial pressure of nitrogen equals 78 percent of 14.7 psi, or 11.6 psi.

A reaction to oxygen, sometimes referred to as oxygen toxicity, can occur when the partial pressure of oxygen equals 1.6 atmospheres absolute, or 23.5 psi (1.6 times 14.7 psi). This could happen if you were breathing pure oxygen (not air) at a depth of just under 20 feet. It could also happen by breathing compressed air at a depth of 250 feet, or 8.6 atmospheres (8.6 times 3.09 psi) (Fig. 9-2).

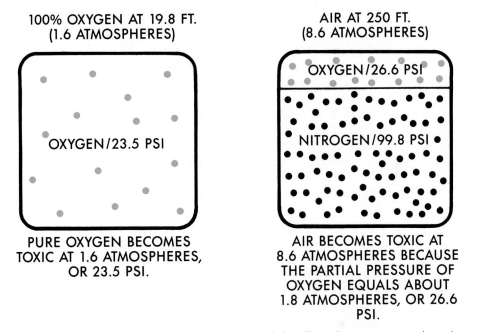

100% OXYGEN AT 19.8 FT.
(1.6 ATMOSPHERES)

OXYGEN/23.5 PSI

PURE OXYGEN BECOMES
TOXIC AT 1.6 ATMOSPHERES,
OR 23.5 PSI.

AIR AT 250 FT.
(8.6 ATMOSPHERES)

OXYGEN/26.6 PSI

NITROGEN/99.8 PSI

AIR BECOMES TOXIC AT
8.6 ATMOSPHERES BECAUSE
THE PARTIAL PRESSURE OF
OXYGEN EQUALS ABOUT
1.8 ATMOSPHERES, OR 26.6
PSI.

Fig. 9-2 *Illustration of the concentration of gases and the effect of pressure. Note that when oxygen becomes 26.2 psi at 8.6 ATA, there is a risk of a toxic reaction to oxygen.*

An adverse reaction to oxygen—oxygen toxicity—will never be a problem for the sport diver who uses clean, dry, filtered air only and stays within the 100-foot depth limit for sport diving.

Symptoms of an oxygen reaction are muscular twitching, nausea, vision and hearing problems, breathing difficulties, anxiety, confusion, unusual fatigue, clumsiness, and seizures. These symptoms stop as soon as the partial pressure of oxygen is reduced below 14.7 psi either by decreasing ambient pressure or by reducing the concentration of oxygen in the breathing mixture. Oxygen toxicity underwater usually leads to drowning.

DECOMPRESSION SICKNESS

The nitrogen in the diver's compressed breathing air is responsible for decompression sickness as well as nitrogen narcosis. Decompression sickness (DCS), or the bends as it is called, is certainly the most notorious of diving illnesses. The story of the diver crippled with the "bends," yet saved in the nick of time by a recompression chamber, has provided suspense and drama to more than one diving movie. *Decompression sickness is as serious a diving ailment as air embolism—they are both life-threatening.*

Decompression sickness was identified in the nineteenth century among French workers building supports for a bridge across the Loire River. They worked in 65-foot shafts, called caissons, which were pressurized to keep water from seeping in. At the end of every 7-hour work day under pressure, the workers returned to atmospheric pressure on the surface. Two of the workers developed pain in their joints. Their symptoms became known as "caisson disease." Later cases reported among workers and sponge divers found some of the patients being bent over with their pain and others seemingly choking. The terms "bends" and "chokes" were coined to additionally describe the disease.

In 1878, Paul Bert identified nitrogen as the agent responsible for the disease and stated that nitrogen bubbles forming in tissues following exposure to increased gas pressures and subsequent decompression were the probable cause of the symptoms. In this sense, decompression means to reduce the pressure—the opposite of compression.

The first decompression tables were developed by Haldane, Boycott, and Damant in Great Britain to limit time under pressure to avoid DCS. The researchers proposed a theory of tissue saturation with nitrogen and established the basic concepts upon which current decompression tables are based. Those concepts included stage decompression, which is done in steps (stages) at specified depths beneath the surface. The stage decompression process helps a diver avoid decompression sickness by allowing excess nitrogen to escape from the body through respiration instead of by forming small nitrogen bubbles in the blood and tissues.

According to Henry's Law, gases will dissolve in a liquid in proportion to the partial pressure of the gas on the liquid. If you double the partial pressure of nitrogen, for example, the amount of nitrogen that can dissolve in the blood and tissues of the body also doubles. If you triple the pressure, blood and tissues can hold three times the amount of nitrogen.

Nitrogen dissolved in the body is harmless as long as it stays dissolved. Nitrogen, oxygen, carbon dioxide, and other gases transfer into and out of the bloodstream via the alveoli of the lungs constantly, whether you are diving or not. However, if you reduce the ambient pressure too quickly, the dissolved nitrogen comes out of solution in the form of tiny bubbles in the blood and tissues of the body.

The classic example of dissolved gas coming out of solution is a soda pop bottle, shown in Fig. 9-3. With the cap on, no bubbles are visible because the liquid is under pressure, and the carbonization bubbles (carbon dioxide gas) are held in solution or are too small to be seen. When you take the cap off, the pressure is suddenly reduced. The soda bubbles, with bubbles seeming to come from nowhere but actually coming from the soda itself as the gas is released from solution. The soda will continue to bubble until it goes "flat." A flat bottle of soda does not bubble because the partial pressure of carbon dioxide gas dissolved in the liquid equals the partial pressure of the gas at ambient pressure—the air surrounding the liquid.

A bubbling, carbonated beverage decompresses in much the same way that liq-

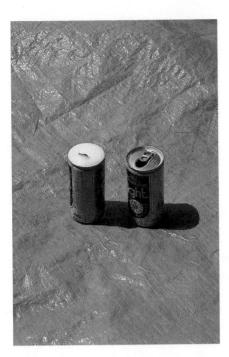

Fig. 9-3 *The beer can shown foaming here, demonstrates how bubbles might form in human tissues. If the gas is coming out of solution faster than it can be directly absorbed in the atmosphere, bubbles form. In the other can, the gas is escaping more slowly and foam (bubbles) are not visible.*

uids and tissues of the body decompress during decompression sickness. To avoid this active bubbling, then, you remove the cap slowly; to avoid decompression sickness, decompress slowly by staying well within the recommended limits and using proper ascent rates.

The symptoms of decompression sickness vary, depending on where the nitrogen bubbles form in the body. Additionally, the process of the body's reaction to nitrogen bubbles is such that problems associated with the disease go far beyond the simple formation of bubbles to include clotting, reduction of circulating blood volume, and other dramatic physiological changes.

Symptoms

Symptoms of decompression sickness usually develop more than 10 minutes after but will probably occur within the first hour after a diver surfaces. Symptoms have been reported as late as 36 hours after the exposure to pressure.

Some common signs and symptoms of decompression sickness include joint pain, skin rash, numbness and tingling in the extremities, personality change, fatigue, impairment of vision, and weakness. More severe signs and symptoms can include paralysis, blindness, seizures, and unconsciousness.

Prevention

The U.S. Navy has set up a no-decompression limits table listing the number of minutes at which you can stay at certain depths and theoretically still avoid decompression sickness after returning directly to the surface. The U.S. Navy table is reproduced in the Appendix and includes depth-time limits as follows:

35 feet—310 minutes
40 feet—200 minutes
50 feet—100 minutes
60 feet— 60 minutes
70 feet— 50 minutes
80 feet— 40 minutes
90 feet— 30 minutes
100 feet— 25 minutes

Even if you abide strictly by these limits, however, avoidance of DCS cannot be guaranteed. One reason is that the U.S. Navy diving tables are based on the diving experiences of a group of trained, healthy military men, whereas sport divers range widely in physical condition and ability.

Several factors reduce the effectiveness of the no-decompression limits table. Basically, any factor that alters normal blood circulation can change the limits. These factors include age, fatigue, the use of alcohol or drugs, old injuries, dehydration, hot showers after diving, and even tightly fitting dive suits.

Obesity also makes a diver more susceptible to decompression sickness. Fat absorbs about five times as much nitrogen as muscle. Though it takes longer for fatty tissues to become saturated with nitrogen, it also takes longer for the nitrogen to leave these tissues during decompression.

It is felt that the use of birth control pills makes a woman diver more susceptible to decompression sickness because of the pills' effects on her body. Though not quantified, the possibility of an increased risk can be easily offset by conservative calculations done with the dive tables.

Pregnancy, because of the harm even undetectable decompression sickness could possibly cause a fetus, is a condition that should keep you from diving. The conservative, and only recommended, approach to diving while pregnant is to abstain altogether.

It is important to note that even though the no-decompression limits table indicates that you can dive as long as you wish at certain depths, it is best to avoid extreme exposures even at shallow depths. As a general rule, be more conservative than indicated in the table (e.g., many divers subtract 5 minutes from each no-decompression limit duration when planning their dive or limit their dives to within two pressure groups of the no-decompression limit).

Ascent Rate

Every decompression table developed prescribes the rate at which you should ascend. The U.S. Navy standard air decompression table has an ascent rate of 60 feet per minute maximum. However, many tables and agencies now recommend that the ascent rate be limited to no more than 40 feet per minute, and a slower rate is preferable. Some diving computer manufacturers are building ascent rates of 15 feet per minute into their computer program with audible and visual warnings when limits are exceeded. Sport divers have a tendency to ascend too rapidly;

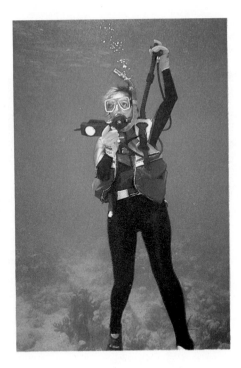

Fig. 9-4 *Ascend at the rate recommended by the tables you are following or slower.*

therefore, whatever the recommended ascent rate of the table you utilize may be, for your own safety, do not exceed the ascent rate recommended (Fig. 9-4).

Recognizing that this book will be utilized by many instructors who follow a variety of tables, no recommendations favoring one table over another are made, but you should fully comply with any limits advocated by whatever table you are taught to use. Don't switch tables or computers while doing multiple dives.

Table Selection

Throughout this text, we utilize the U.S. Navy standard air decompression tables, as they remain the tested standard in sport scuba diving. However, the Appendix contains a table which compares those of the U.S. Navy, the DCIEM, PADI, and NAUI.

Bottom Time

In the U.S. Navy tables, the no-decompression limits are given in minutes of bottom time for the deepest depth reached. To use the tables, you consider yourself "on the bottom" from the time you begin your descent until the time you begin your ascent directly to the surface, as illustrated in Fig. 9-5. For example, if you descend to 25 feet for 10 minutes, then continue deeper to 50 feet for 15 minutes, after which you ascend back to 25 feet for 5 minutes, and then ascend directly to the surface, your "bottom time" is 30 minutes at 50 feet, even though you spent only 15 minutes at 50 feet.

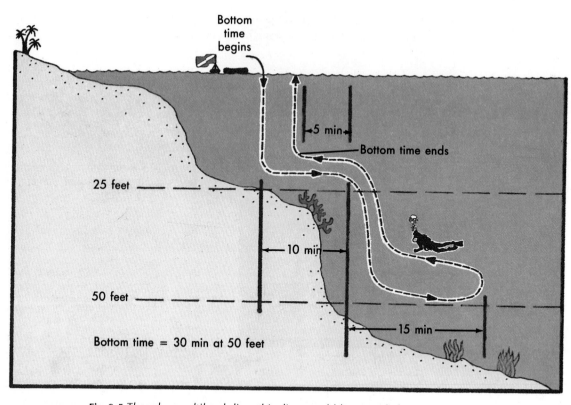

Fig. 9-5 *Though a multilevel dive, this dive would be recorded as 30 minutes at 50 feet.*

Bottom time refers to the *total* time of the dive from the beginning of the descent to the beginning of the final direct ascent to the surface. The depth of the dive, when using tables, is always the deepest point of the dive, no matter how briefly you stay at that depth.

In addition, if your time or depth is not listed exactly in the tables, you must go up to the next higher time or next greater depth respectively. *Do not round to the nearest value* but always round to the more conservative time or depth. Bottom time and depth are also discussed in Chapter 10.

ALTITUDE DIVING

Diving in mountain lakes or other high-altitude waters increases the possibility of decompression sickness, unless you utilize dive tables specifically intended for increased altitude. The U.S. Navy decompression tables, for instance, are not to be used at altitudes over 2,300 feet above sea level. When you ascend from a dive at a high altitude location, the atmospheric pressure is lower than at sea level. This results in a greater difference between water pressures at depth and air pressures at the surface. Because of this, some decompression computers and depth gauges are inaccurate above sea level. If you plan to dive at high altitudes, you should use a set of high-altitude dive tables that have been approved by your certification agency.

FLYING AFTER DIVING

Flying after diving increases your susceptibility to DCS because of the decreased atmospheric pressure at high altitude. Airplanes are usually pressurized above sea level pressures (usually 6,000 to 8,500 feet), and this can cause serious decompression problems for a diver partially saturated with nitrogen. Though most tables and agencies still permit flying 12 hours after your final dive, diving accident statistics may lead to the conclusion that you should wait for at least 24 hours before flying after any diving. If you have done multiday, multilevel diving, the same information may lead you to wait more than 24 hours after your last dive before flying.

TREATMENT OF DECOMPRESSION SICKNESS

Currently, the most effective treatment of decompression sickness is immediate recompression in a recompression chamber. See Fig. 9-6 for a look into a chamber. Recompression reduces the size of the nitrogen bubbles and forces them back into solution. Combining oxygen with pressure, the partial pressure of oxygen in the body increases and tends to drive nitrogen out of the body as well as increasing oxygen flow to those tissues that might have been damaged by the decompression sickness. Then pressure is gradually decreased to allow the diver to decompress slowly without the formation of new nitrogen bubbles.

At the first sign of possible symptoms of decompression sickness, seek treatment immediately. First aid before reaching a recompression chamber is identical to that outlined for air embolism described in Chapter 8.

The emergency plan you develop before diving should include where to go for

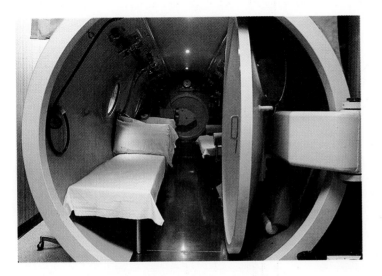

Fig. 9-6 *An inside look at a recompression chamber.*

recompression in the event of an accident in which decompression sickness or air embolism is suspected.

If you have an accident and do not know where to go for recompression, call Divers Alert Network (DAN) at 919-684-8111. In an emergency, DAN will accept collect calls and can be called from anywhere in the United States, the Caribbean, or the Gulf of Mexico. Underwater recompression should not be considered because of the danger in the event of unconsciousness, seizures, and other ill effects that might be associated with DCS.

SUMMARY

The indirect effects of pressure can be easily avoided by setting safe depth and time limits for your sport diving. Since most underwater life lives well within the warm and lighted depths above 100 feet, dive there and keep your diving enjoyable, interesting, and safe.

10 Repetitive Dives

- Residual Nitrogen
- Repetitive Diving
- Dive Profile
- Decompression Diving

At the conclusion of Chapter 10, you will be able to:

1. Tell how long it takes for the body to become saturated with nitrogen.
2. State how saturated nitrogen is released from the body.
3. Explain why divers complete dive profiles after a dive.
4. Define "surface interval."
5. Explain the difference between actual and total bottom times.
6. Explain what is meant by a repetitive dive.
7. State the surface interval between dives that would cause two dives to be treated as a long single dive.
8. State the length of time that must elapse before you can assume there is no more residual nitrogen, according to the U.S. Navy tables.
9. Name the type of diving not appropriate for sport diving but about which you should be familiar for safety's sake.

KEY TERMS

Saturated	Bottom time	Depth
Surface interval time	Repetitive dive	Group
RNT	ABT	TBT
SIT	NDL	ANDL

Residual Nitrogen, More Than One Dive, and Decompression Diving
RESIDUAL NITROGEN

Your body normally contains an amount of nitrogen dissolved in the blood and tissues that is in equilibrium with the surrounding ambient pressure. Whenever you dive, your body starts to absorb more nitrogen because of the increased pressure underwater. The blood and tissues will continue to absorb nitrogen for about 24 hours under the new pressure. After 24 hours, the body is said to be saturated with nitrogen—the N_2 pressure inside the body equals the N_2 pressure in the environment, so absorption stops.

When you return to the lower pressure at the surface, the nitrogen slowly leaves the blood and tissues through normal respiration via the alveoli in the lungs. The body continues to release nitrogen until the extra gas dissolved in blood and tissues is gone and the body is back to its normal surface equilibrium, usually within about 12 hours.

The extra nitrogen that is in your body after a dive is called "residual nitrogen."

Decompression tables are more or less based on the simple fact that the residual nitrogen will stay in solution and not form bubbles as long as the partial pressure of nitrogen is not immediately reduced by more than 45 percent to 55 percent. Studies have indicated that very small bubbles may be formed and remain in the blood even if a diver stays within the no-decompression limits of a dive table. Provided they remain in the venous circulation, these bubbles are thought to be harmless and are eventually filtered out by the lungs. If these bubbles, even though they may be quite small, end up in arterial circulation, however, they can cause very serious problems.

Considering this, it is recommended that you do not dive to the maximum limits of a no-decompression table, in order to decrease the possibility of developing decompression sickness (see Chapter 9). As an added safety measure, it is prudent for you to stop at 15 feet from the surface for at least 3 minutes after every no-decompression dive.

MORE THAN ONE DIVE

The no-decompression limits and repetitive group designation tables for no-decompression air dives indicate how long you can stay at certain depths in *salt water* and yet return to the surface without decompression stops.

What if you want to make another dive soon after the first one? Since your body contains some residual nitrogen from the first dive, you will not be able to stay as long on your second dive, as you otherwise might, before you reach the limit. The tables outlined in the Appendix, when used correctly, help you to figure the time effect your residual nitrogen has on a subsequent dive.

A Typical Repetitive Dive

Fig. 10-1 is a diagram of two dives. A buddy team plans to make a dive in the morning and one after lunch. They descend at 11 AM to a maximum depth of 73 feet and swim along the bottom toward the shore. The bottom becomes slightly shal-

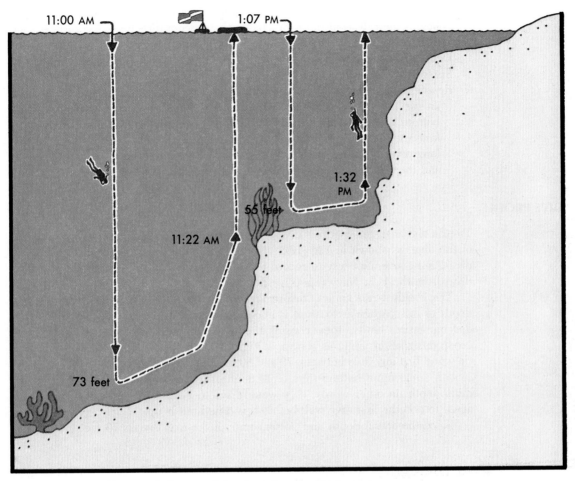

Fig. 10-1 *A diagram of the dives described in the text.*

lower as they swim, until they run into a vertical underwater cliff. They ascend along the face of the cliff until they discover an underwater ledge at 55 feet. After finding the ledge, they agree to ascend as planned. They both note the time as 11:22 AM and begin a direct ascent to the surface, stopping at 15 feet for a 2-minute safety stop.

After eating lunch and refilling their cylinders, the buddy team begins their descent at 1:07 PM. They explore the underwater ledge at a depth of 55 feet for 25 minutes. At 1:32 PM, they start their ascent from 55 feet to the surface, again stopping for a 2-minute safety stop.

Before, during, and after these two dives, the buddy team used the U.S. Navy tables to plan and recheck both the time and the depth of each dive. To use and understand the table, you should become familiar with several important terms:

Bottom time refers to the total elapsed time starting from when the buddy team begins their descent until they begin their ascent directly to the surface. (See Chapter 9.)

Depth is the deepest point reached during a dive.

Surface interval time is the length of time on the surface between dives.

Repetitive dive refers to any dive that begins within 12 hours of surfacing from an earlier dive. This applies to most sport dives. If you accumulate a lot of bottom time, take longer surface intervals than the tables require. If the surface interval between dives is 10 minutes or less, consider both dives as one long dive, with a bottom time equal to the total bottom times of both dives and the depth being the deepest depth reached on either dive.

DIVE PROFILE

To plan and analyze repetitive dives more easily, the buddy team sketches a profile of the dive, as shown in Fig. 10-2. The profile, a simple diagram of one or more dives, is a convenient way to record time, depth, and information about repetitive dives from the U.S. Navy repetitive dive tables.

The buddy team knows, before arriving at the dive site, that the maximum depth of this particular location is about 75 feet. In order to stay within the no-decompression limits, they consult the no-decompression limits and repetitive group designation table, as shown in Fig. 10-3. Looking at the first two columns, they find that any dive between 70 and 80 feet is considered a dive to 80 feet (Item 1) with a maximum bottom time of 40 minutes (Item 2). If they went to the maximum depth, in other words, they would have to ascend within 40 minutes. They agree to end the first dive well before this time limit is up.

Since the actual depth and bottom time of the first dive is 73 feet for 22 min-

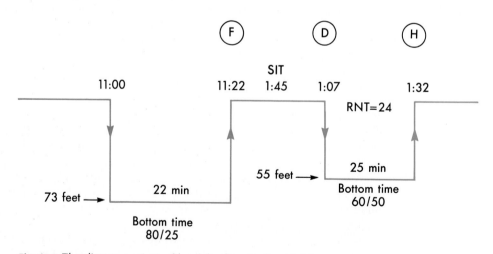

Fig. 10-2 *The diagrammatic profile of the dive in Fig. 10-1 is an easy way to record information regarding the dive as well as to plan repetitive dives.*

NO-DECOMPRESSION LIMITS AND REPETITIVE GROUP DESIGNATION TABLE FOR NO-DECOMPRESSION AIR DIVES

Group Designation [4] → F

Depth (feet)	No-decompression limits (min)	A	B	C	D	E	F	G	H	I	J	K	L	M	N	O
10		60	120	210	300											
15	[1]	35	70	110	160	225	350									
20		25	50	75	100	135	180	240	325							
25	(245)	20	35	55	75	100	125	160	195	245	315					
30	(205)	15	30	45	60	75	95	120	145	170	205	250	310			
35	(160) 310	5	15	25	40	50	60	80	100	120	140	160	190	220	270	310
40	(130) 200	5	15	25	30	40	50	70	80	100	110	130	150	170	200	
50	(70) 100		10	15	25	30	40	50	60	70	80	90	100			
60	(50) 60 [2]		10	15	20	25	30	40	50	55	60					
70	(40) 50		5	10	15	20	30	35	40	45	50					
80	(30) 40		5	10	15	20	25	30	35	40						
90	(25) 30		5	10	12	15	20	25	30							
100	(20) 25		5	7	10	15	20	22	25							
110	(15) 20			5	10	13	15	20								
120	(10) 15			5	10	12	15									
130	(5) 10			5	8	10	[3]									
140	10			5	7	10										

Fig. 10-3 *No-decompression limits table.*

utes, they enter this information on the dive profile. Returning to the no-decompression table for the 80-foot depth, they find that the *exact or next greater* time, over 22 minutes, is 25 minutes (Item 3). They next enter this information in the profile: "80/25."

The shaded area in Fig. 10-3 illustrates that a dive to 80 feet for 25 minutes puts the dive team in repetitive group "F" (Item 4). They enter this information in the dive profile. The repetitive groups "A" through "O" actually represent a system for cataloging how much residual nitrogen remains in a diver's body after a no-decompression dive. An "A" diver, for example, has very little residual nitrogen, while an "O" diver has a great amount.

The surface interval time between dives is 1 hour and 45 minutes. They enter this time in the dive profile. While the buddy team is on the surface, they are constantly giving off nitrogen. When they begin the repetitive dive, therefore, their bodies contain less residual nitrogen than they did at the end of the first dive. To get credit for this decrease in residual nitrogen, they turn to the second table, the residual nitrogen timetable for repetitive air dives, as shown in Fig. 10-4.

Since the dive team ended the first dive as "F" divers, they enter the residual nitrogen timetable at "F" on the slanted left-hand side of the table. The paired numbers, to the right, refer to the minimum and maximum surface interval times.

Reading from left to right (Fig. 10-5), they find that their time, 1 hour and 45 minutes, puts them in the fourth column from the right side of the table, or the box containing 1:30 (minimum time in that designation) and 2:28 (maximum time). Following the column downward, the buddies find they have given off residual nitrogen to move from the "F" group designation to the "D" group designation.

The buddy team has less residual nitrogen in their bodies, but they still have

RESIDUAL NITROGEN TIMETABLE FOR REPETITIVE AIR DIVES

*Dives following surface intervals of more than 12 hours are not repetitive dives. Use actual bottom times in the Standard Air Decompression Tables to compute decompression for such dives.

Repetitive group at the beginning of the surface interval

Repetitive group	Z	O	N	M	L	K	J	I	H	G	F	E	D	C	B	A
A																0:10–12:00*
B															0:10–2:10	2:11–12:00*
C														0:10–1:39	1:40–2:49	2:50–12:00*
D													0:10–1:09	1:10–2:38	2:39–5:48	5:49–12:00*
E												0:10–0:54	0:55–1:57	1:58–3:22	3:23–6:32	6:33–12:00*
F											0:10–0:45	0:46–1:29	1:30–2:28	2:29–3:57	3:58–7:05	7:06–12:00*
G										0:10–0:40	0:41–1:15	1:16–1:59	2:00–2:58	2:59–4:25	4:26–7:35	7:36–12:00*
H									0:10–0:36	0:37–1:06	1:07–1:41	1:42–2:23	2:24–3:20	3:21–4:49	4:50–7:59	8:00–12:00*
I								0:10–0:33	0:34–0:59	1:00–1:29	1:30–2:02	2:03–2:44	2:45–3:43	3:44–5:12	5:13–8:21	8:22–12:00*
J							0:10–0:31	0:32–0:54	0:55–1:19	1:20–1:47	1:48–2:20	2:21–3:04	3:05–4:02	4:03–5:40	5:41–8:40	8:41–12:00*
K						0:10–0:28	0:29–0:49	0:50–1:11	1:12–1:35	1:36–2:03	2:04–2:38	2:39–3:21	3:22–4:19	4:20–5:48	5:49–8:58	8:59–12:00*
L					0:10–0:26	0:27–0:45	0:46–1:04	1:05–1:25	1:26–1:49	1:50–2:19	2:20–2:53	2:54–3:36	3:37–4:35	4:36–6:02	6:03–9:12	9:13–12:00*
M				0:10–0:25	0:26–0:42	0:43–0:59	1:00–1:18	1:19–1:39	1:40–2:05	2:06–2:34	2:35–3:08	3:09–3:52	3:53–4:49	4:50–6:18	6:19–9:28	9:29–12:00*
N			0:10–0:24	0:25–0:39	0:40–0:54	0:55–1:11	1:12–1:30	1:31–1:53	1:54–2:18	2:19–2:47	2:48–3:22	3:23–4:04	4:05–5:03	5:04–6:32	6:33–9:43	9:44–12:00*
O		0:10–0:23	0:24–0:36	0:37–0:51	0:52–1:07	1:08–1:24	1:25–1:43	1:44–2:04	2:05–2:29	2:30–2:59	3:00–3:33	3:34–4:17	4:18–5:16	5:17–6:44	6:45–9:54	9:55–12:00*
Z	0:10–0:22	0:23–0:34	0:35–0:48	0:49–1:02	1:03–1:18	1:19–1:36	1:37–1:55	1:56–2:17	2:18–2:42	2:43–3:10	3:11–3:45	3:46–4:29	4:30–5:27	5:28–6:56	6:57–10:05	10:06–12:00*

NEW GROUP DESIGNATION →

REPETITIVE DIVE DEPTH	Z	O	N	M	L	K	J	I	H	G	F	E	D	C	B	A
40	257	241	213	187	161	138	116	101	87	73	61	49	37	25	17	7
50	169	160	142	124	111	99	87	76	66	56	47	38	29	21	13	6
60	122	117	107	97	88	79	70	61	52	44	36	30	24	17	11	5
70	100	96	87	80	72	64	57	50	43	37	31	26	20	15	9	4
80	84	80	73	68	61	54	48	43	38	32	28	23	18	13	8	4
90	73	70	64	58	53	47	43	38	33	29	24	20	16	11	7	3
100	64	62	57	52	48	43	38	34	30	26	22	18	14	10	7	3
110	57	55	51	47	42	38	34	31	27	24	20	16	13	10	6	3
120	52	50	46	43	39	35	32	28	25	21	18	15	12	9	6	3
130	46	44	40	38	35	31	28	25	22	19	16	13	11	8	6	3
140	42	40	38	35	32	29	26	23	20	18	15	12	10	7	5	2
150	40	38	35	32	30	27	24	22	19	17	14	12	9	7	5	2
160	37	36	33	31	28	26	23	20	18	16	13	11	9	6	4	2
170	35	34	31	29	26	24	22	19	17	15	13	10	8	6	4	2
180	32	31	29	27	25	22	20	18	16	14	12	10	8	6	4	2
190	31	30	28	26	24	21	19	17	15	13	11	10	8	6	4	2

RESIDUAL NITROGEN TIMES (MINUTES)

Fig. 10-4 Residual nitrogen timetable.

some nitrogen that must be taken into account for the second dive. The new group designation letter "D" is added to the dive profile. Then, they turn to the lower half of the residual nitrogen timetable shown in Fig. 10-4. The purpose of this part of the table is to convert the group letter and the depth of the next repetitive dive into minutes of residual nitrogen time, which the buddy team must consider that they have already spent on the bottom *before* they begin the next repetitive dive. Depths for the next dive are listed in the far left-hand column.

The shaded area in Fig. 10-5 shows that a "D" diver going to a repetitive dive depth of 60 feet will have a residual nitrogen time of 24 minutes. The residual nitrogen time (RNT) is added to the dive profile. This means that our buddy team

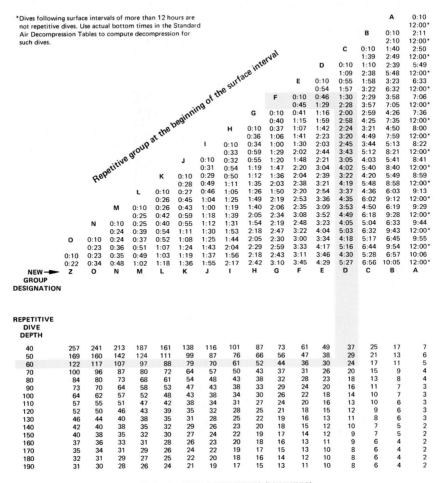

RESIDUAL NITROGEN TIMETABLE FOR REPETITIVE AIR DIVES

Fig. 10-5 *Residual nitrogen timetable.*

must *start* their second dive to 55 feet as though they had already been at this depth for 24 minutes.

Now, to make sure that they do not go beyond the no-decompression limits, they go back to the no-decompression limits table (Fig. 10-6) and find that a dive to 60 feet (55 actual feet) will have a maximum bottom time of 60 minutes.

In order to stay well within the no-decompression limits, the buddy team decides to limit their actual bottom time to 25 minutes. Since they are beginning the repetitive dive with a residual nitrogen time of 24 minutes, their total bottom time will be 25 minutes plus 24 minutes, or 49 minutes. This is 11 minutes short of the U.S. Navy no-decompression limit.

NO-DECOMPRESSION LIMITS AND REPETITIVE GROUP DESIGNATION TABLE FOR NO-DECOMPRESSION AIR DIVES

Depth (feet)	No-decompression limits (min)	A	B	C	D	E	F	G	H	I	J	K	L	M	N	O
10		60	120	210	300											
15		35	70	110	160	225	350									
20		25	50	75	100	135	180	240	325							
25	(245)	20	35	55	75	100	125	160	195	245	315					
30	(205)	15	30	45	60	75	95	120	145	170	205	250	310			
35	(160) 310	5	15	25	40	50	60	80	100	120	140	160	190	220	270	310
40	(130) 200	5	15	25	30	40	50	70	80	100	110	130	150	170	200	
50	(70) 100		10	15	25	30	40	50	60	70	80	90	100			
60	(50) 60		10	15	20	25	30	40	50	55	60					
70	(40) 50		5	10	15	20	30	35	40	45	50					
80	(30) 40		5	10	15	20	25	30	35	40						
90	(25) 30		5	10	12	15	20	25	30							
100	(20) 25		5	7	10	15	20	22	25							
110	(15) 20			5	10	13	15	20								
120	(10) 15			5	10	12	15									
130	(5) 10			5	8	10										
140	10			5	7	10										

Group Designation

Fig. 10-6 *No-decompression limits table.*

At the end of the repetitive dive, the two divers use the no-decompression limits table to find their repetitive dive group designation, as shown in Fig. 10-6.

The shaded area in the table shows that their second dive of the day was to 60 feet for 50 minutes (55 actual feet and 49 actual minutes) which makes them "H" divers. The "H" repetitive dive group designation is entered in the profile at the appropriate place where it can be used for another repetitive dive if they decide to make one.

DECOMPRESSION DIVING

Decompression diving—diving longer than the no-decompression limits allow—is not recommended for sport divers. Information relative to decompression stops is included in diving tables used by sport scuba divers not as a dive planning tool but to provide the diver with necessary "stop" information should a diver exceed the prescribed depth-time limits of the table inadvertently.

Good planning and intelligent, accurate use of the repetitive dive tables should almost eliminate the problem of decompression sickness from your diving.

AIDS TO DIVE PLANNING

Dive tables come in a variety of sizes, shapes, and construction, and are based on a wide variety of underlying theories. In this book we have chosen to use the U.S. Navy tables for illustration purposes (Fig. 10-7). However, you may learn to dive using the PADI, NAUI, DCIEM sport diving tables, a "wheel," or some other of the many tables utilized throughout the world. All these tables are created to help you control the amount of saturated nitrogen in your blood and become a safe, intelligent diver.

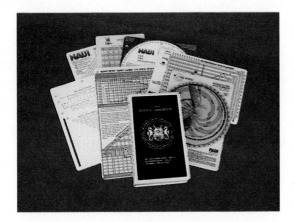

Fig. 10-7 *Whatever dive table you choose to use, make sure you are totally familiar with it.*

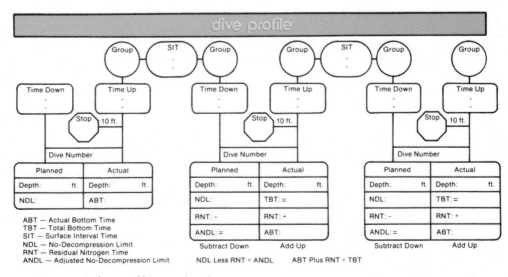

ABT — Actual Bottom Time			
TBT — Total Bottom Time			
SIT — Surface Interval Time			
NDL — No-Decompression Limit			
RNT — Residual Nitrogen Time			
ANDL — Adjusted No-Decompression Limit			

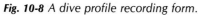

Fig. 10-8 *A dive profile recording form.*

If you are diving with the aid of a table, it is often helpful to use some simplified dive profile recording form such as the one illustrated in Fig. 10-8. This profile form utilizes the "fill-in-the-blanks" approach to record dive information and provides appropriate cues to help you make the necessary calculations.

SUMMARY

As human beings, we have limitations imposed on us underwater by the nitrogen in the compressed air we breathe there. Our intelligence has allowed us to define these limitations and provided us with a system for staying within them yet having time to appreciate and enjoy the underwater world.

Now, all we need is the common sense to abide by our limitations so we can return again and again to our adventures in inner space.

11 The Worlds of Diving

- History of the Oceans
- Ecology
- Environmental Variation
- Weather

At the conclusion of Chapter 11, you will be able to:

1. State the percentage of the earth's surface covered with oceans.
2. State the lowest temperature corals can tolerate.
3. Define the term thermocline.
4. Explain the characteristics of a continental shelf.
5. Name the branch of science which studies the interrelationships of living organisms and their environment.
6. Name the great brown algae that thrive along the colder coasts of North and South America.
7. State whether warm or cold water produces a greater *quantity* of marine life.
8. Explain how to obtain weather information when on board a dive boat.
9. Name the federal agency responsible for weather information.
10. Explain how a front is formed.

KEY TERMS

Icecaps	Continental drift	Ecosystem
Phytoplankton	Thermocline	Overturn
Upwelling	Airmass	NOAA

The oceans cover 70.8 percent of the earth's surface. Thousands of freshwater lakes and rivers contribute even more to the earth's liquid surface. Because of this, astronomers often call earth the "water planet." Earth is definitely the best planet in our solar system for sport divers.

Thinkers and philosophers have long attempted to unravel the mystery of how this planet was blessed with water, but it remains largely unsolved. We know that earth lies just far enough from the sun to prevent the seas from boiling away into a giant cloud surrounding the planet, but it also lies close enough to prevent most of our water from freezing into a big block of ice.

HISTORY OF THE OCEANS

Attempts at solving some of the mysteries of the oceans began as early as 2 BC. Posidonius wrote that a depth of 1,000 fathoms had been measured in the Sea of Sardinia, but study of the oceans did not become a separate branch of science until the nineteenth century.

Despite the remarkable advances made in oceanography in the last century and a half, controversy about how the water entered the oceans still remains. Some geologists think that all of primeval earth's water existed as atmospheric vapor, which condensed and fell in great torrents when the earth cooled. Others hold that water gradually accumulated when volcanoes released it as steam or when it came to the surface in hot springs.

We may not know the origin of the water on the earth's crust, but we do know that about 85 percent of it is now in the oceans. The rest is found inland and frozen in the polar icecaps.

Compared to continental land, relatively little is known about the land beneath the ocean. Growing evidence indicates that the rocks underlying the ocean floors are more dense than those underlying the continents. According to the continental drift theory, the earth's crust floats on a central liquid core. The continents, being lighter, float with a higher freeboard and are slowly drifting apart. Other areas, composed of heavier rock, form natural basins where water has collected.

Along most of the continents' coasts, the bottom gradually slopes down to about

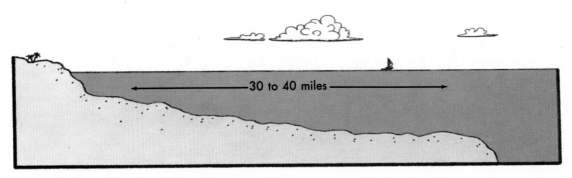

Fig. 11-1 Continental shelf.

600 feet (183 meters), after which it falls away more rapidly to greater depths. The continental shelf, as shown in Fig. 11-1, averages about 30 miles in width, but can vary from zero to about 800 miles. A similar shelf usually extends out from islands or groups of islands.

In general, the deep sea bottom slopes gradually, averaging about half a degree. But it may slope as much as 45 degrees off a volcanic island, and sometimes it drops almost straight down. The topography of the ocean bottom looks a lot like the continents. Both have steep, rugged mountains, deep canyons, rolling hills, and plains.

ECOLOGY

Ecology is the branch of science that studies the interrelationships of living organisms and their environment. The underwater ecosystem is so intimately interrelated that it is sometimes difficult to distinguish living organisms from their environment; the fish is in the sea, but the sea is also in the fish. Perhaps we could think of the sea as a living broth, or even as a single infinitely complex, living organism.

Seawater not only has all the chemical elements needed to sustain life, it also has about 300 times more living space than dry land. As a result, the sea contains vast quantities of organic material such as nutrients, plants, and animals.

The underwater plants and animals are so dependent on each other and on their environment that if we destroy any major link in this intricate food chain, or if we poison the environment and thus kill any part of this cycle of life, then we must face the real and frightening possibility of all the world's oceans becoming a giant dead sea with no life to enjoy or no life to help keep us land animals alive. Pollution and other threats to the underwater ecosystem are discussed in Chapter 15.

ENVIRONMENTAL VARIATION

An overview of the diving environment usually gives the impression that all parts of the entire underwater world with its basins and life cycles are basically the same. In some respects this is true. A small wave breaking on a pond's shore in Minnesota and an enormous breaker crashing on the shore of Australia both obey the same laws. But a closer look reveals endless variations in application of these laws.

The variables include bottom types, currents, plant and animal life, color and transparency, and a host of others that depend on time and place. All these variables, however, have something in common. In almost all cases, they either depend on, or are closely associated with, differences in temperature.

Temperature

Geology dictates basic bottom types such as rock, mud, or sand, but water temperature gives a dive site its distinctive life.

Reef-building corals, for example, flourish in tropical and subtropical areas on the eastern shores of continents where the sea's mean annual temperature is at least 74.3° F (23.5° C), as shown in Fig. 11-2. Most corals cannot withstand water temperatures much below 64° F (18° C).

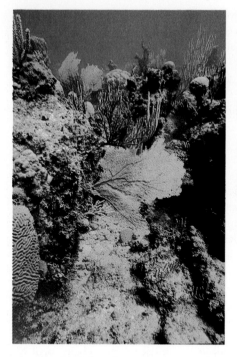

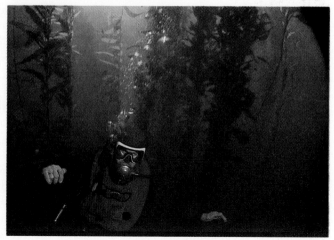

Fig. 11-3 Kelp found in colder water.

Fig. 11-2 A coral reef.

Along the colder coasts of North and South America, on the other hand, the great brown algae known as kelp thrive, as shown in Fig. 11-3.

The amount of marine life in the water also depends on water temperature, although the relationship is an indirect one. The amount of marine life is directly related to the supply of phytoplankton in the water, and the supply of phytoplankton depends on a good supply of sunlight and chemical nutrients.

In shallow waters, water movement usually stirs up the bottom and carries nutrients to the sunlit surface, so animal life abounds. Life also thrives in polar regions where the water's surface is supplied with nutrients lifted from the bottom by rising warm-water currents.

Surprisingly, the warm water tropics produce relatively little phytoplankton, as chemical nutrients tend to sink in the stable waters below the sunlit surface. As a result, warm waters tend to produce an enormous *variety*, while cold waters tend to produce a great *quantity* of marine life.

The effects of temperature on plants and animals are relatively stable and permanent, but water temperatures at a given location can change dramatically from month to month. Water temperatures range from 85° F (29° C) in the tropics, to 40° F (4° C) at 100 feet in the Great Lakes, to a low of 28° F (−2° C) beneath polar ice. The average temperature of surface water in the ocean is about 63° F (17° C). Surface temperatures vary an average of about 18° F (11° C) during the year.

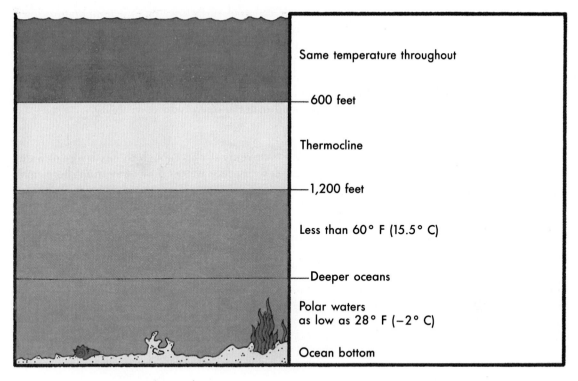

Fig. 11-4 *Thermocline.*

Thermoclines

Thermoclines are layers of water in which the temperature changes significantly, close to the surface or deep in the water. In a thermocline, temperatures can vary 20° F (12° C) or more. With depth, water temperatures decrease nearly everywhere. Colder water, because it is more dense, is usually found below warmer water.

In general, the temperature is the same in the top layer of tropical sea water, which can extend as deep as 600 feet. Below this layer is a zone of rapid temperature decrease called the thermocline, shown in Fig. 11-4. At about 1,200 feet, the temperature may be less than 60° F (15.5° C). Farther below this the deeper layers of the ocean are fed by cooled waters that have sunk from the surface in the Arctic and Antarctic. Temperatures as low as 33° F (0.5° C) exist there.

In northern freshwater lakes, water as cold as 38° F (4° C) can be located at depths of 20 to 30 feet below the thermocline.

Overturns

During the winter and summer months, lakes and oceans usually remain stratified, with definite zones or layers forming above and below the thermocline. Surface water changes in density, however, when temperatures change. Wind or sudden temperature drops in the ambient air can cool surface water to a temperature lower than that of the water immediately below it. When this happens, the surface water sinks to join levels of water having the same temperature, and is replaced by the water just below it.

This water, in turn, may be cooled and will settle, until the rising water is approximately the same temperature as the surrounding air. The cycle then stabilizes. During these overturns, suspended material often reduces visibility.

Upwellings

Strong surface winds can also cause currents strong enough to mix layers of water. A wind blowing off the shore can make surface waters flow away from shore, making colder bottom water flow in to replace them. This phenomenon is called upwelling (see Fig. 11-5). Because the colder, nutrient-rich waters rise from the bottom, upwellings are often associated with huge increases in the plankton population, and corresponding decreases in visibility.

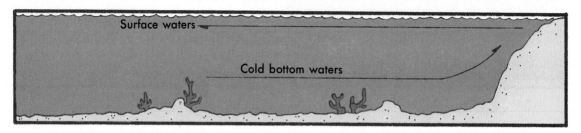

Surface waters

Cold bottom waters

Fig. 11-5 Upwelling.

WEATHER

Along with ecology and environmental variation, weather helps determine the quality of a sport dive. Since most weather is the result of air mass interaction, which can be measured, tracked, and predicted, a short study of air mass interaction and prediction should remove weather as a surprise in our dive planning.

Air Masses

Air masses are large bodies of air with particular temperature, moisture, and barometric pressure characteristics as a result of where and how they were formed. Weather conditions any place are dependent upon either the prevailing air mass, or the interaction between two or more air masses.

Fronts

Air masses with different characteristics do not mix easily, so that when two meet, they form a frontal zone, or front, at their natural boundary. In this frontal zone, weather may change very rapidly or very subtly, often being quite unstable and stormy.

Weather Forecasting

Fortunately for dive-planning purposes, the National Weather Service observes and tracks air masses in order to develop weather forecasts based on their characteristics and interactions. These forecasts are the basis for marine weather reports and broadcasts in coastal areas and around large bodies of water. They also provide information for television weather reports, which often include the details of relevant air masses and frontal activity supported by radar displays showing precipitation and satellite photos of cloud cover. Finally, a forecast of imminent weather is usually provided as well.

Broadcast radio stations also use the National Weather Service to report on present weather and forecasts. Another source of weather information is a special continuous National Oceanic and Atmospheric Administration (NOAA) broadcast on radio throughout the United States and Canada which is localized so as to be pertinent only to the area serviced by the local transmitter. The broadcasts may be received on special weather radios, which can be obtained from home entertainment and electronic stores, or on marine VHF-FM radio weather channels (frequencies 162.550, 162.400, and 162.475). The many sources of weather information are certainly sufficient to provide up-to-date weather information for planning a dive.

Though official weather reports and forecasts are helpful, a smart diver begins to analyze the weather several days before a planned dive. By noting the movement of relevant air masses, developing frontal activity, other significant weather features such as thunderstorms, high water, high waves, or other phenomena which may produce undesirable or dangerous diving conditions, a diver can better evaluate the official reports to determine whether the dive can be conducted as planned.

On the dive day, a diver continues to monitor the weather all the way to the dive site. Rapid cloud build-ups, sudden wind shifts, or temperature changes usually signal deteriorating weather conditions. Continue to listen to radio weather broadcasts and be ready to change your dive plans to avoid bad effects of weather or to benefit from the good.

In some areas, the temperature/dewpoint spread is a significant factor in safe ocean diving. The dewpoint is the temperature to which air must be cooled to become saturated with water vapor. The spread between air temperature and dewpoint therefore indicates how close air is to becoming saturated. When it is small, about 5° F or less, fog should be anticipated, so a smart diver would be sure to have an operable compass for an orderly return to the boat or beach. Likewise, an increase in relative humidity—the amount of water vapor actually in the air—indicates that the air is becoming more and more saturated and fog or precipitation may occur.

A falling barometer also usually indicates a deterioration in weather conditions.

Do not get caught unprepared! No matter where you are in the water, the weather can change dramatically in a very short time. Good weather at the beginning of a dive can turn to bad weather before the end of a dive. Be aware of the weather at all times and conduct your dive accordingly.

DIVING ON THE WATER PLANET

As a sport diver, you should feel fortunate to live on the water planet—the only one in our universe known to have an environment in which to dive. Not only does the environment allow diving, in its many variations, it provides the beauty, vitality, color, and movement that make diving truly magical.

12

Water Movement

- **Tides**
- **Currents**
- **Waves**
- **Surf**
- **Localized Currents**

OBJECTIVES

At the conclusion of Chapter 12, you will be able to:

1. Explain the forces that cause tides.
2. Name the two extremes of tidal movement.
3. State the information provided in tidal current tables.
4. Name three forces that cause ocean currents.
5. Describe how waves are formed.
6. Explain the relationship between fetch and swell.
7. Name the principal risk to a diver entering through a surf.
8. Describe the procedure for doing an entry off a rocky shore.
9. Explain how to make an entry and exit through a coral reef.
10. Describe how a diver might behave if caught in a rip current.

KEY TERMS

High tide	Low tide	Stand
Ebb	Flood	Slack
National Ocean Service	Wind waves	Sea
Swell	Surf zone	Spilling breaker
Plunging breaker	Surging breaker	Longshore current
Rip current		

Tides, Currents, Waves, and Their Effects on Diving

For centuries people have observed the waters of the world with awe. The oceans, in particular, have been a source of inspiration and fear to all who view them. One fear of the oceans stems from misunderstanding the mechanics of water movement. Once you understand the cause and effect of water movement, and once you learn to respect the destructive power of the oceans, you can dive confidently for enjoyment.

If you are an inland diver, with no experience in ocean diving, special instruction will help you dive comfortably in ocean currents and through the surf. Even ocean divers who regularly dive in calm quiet parts of the oceans, such as are found in the tropics, will benefit from specialized training for diving in such places as the cooler waters of New England, kelp forests, or through the west coast surf.

Of course, the same precaution about specialized training applies to ocean divers exploring the hidden excitements and hazards of inland diving in swift rivers, "bottomless" lakes, and wreckage-strewn quarries. This chapter will help you understand water movement and how it can aid you.

TIDES

Among predictable types of worldwide water movement are the tides, which consist of the daily vertical rise and fall of water.

Tides can be thought of as bulges in the water created by the gravitational pull of the moon and sun. When a bulge approaches a given coastline, the water level rises and creates a high tide. As the bulge moves away, the water level drops and low tide results. When the tide changes direction, there is a period in which no vertical motion occurs. This time is referred to as the stand. The tidal range, shown in Fig. 12-1, is the vertical distance between the levels of high and low tides. The tidal flat is the term used to describe the sloping shore that is exposed during low tide.

Generally, divers have an interest in predicting the times of high and low tide. The time of high tide is significant because the water clarity near shore or in bays is

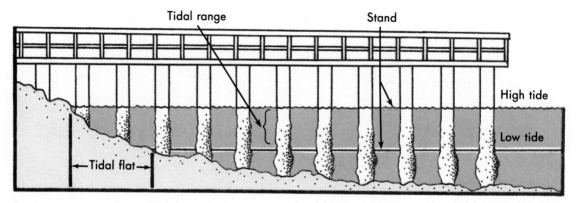

Fig. 12-1 Tidal definitions.

usually best just before high tide because of the influx of clean ocean water. Knowing the time of low tide helps a diver maneuver a boat over shallow spots and it also helps predict a change in surf conditions affected by water depth.

Most dive, fishing, bait, and boat facilities have Tide Tables available which list the times of high and low tides for the local areas.

Since boaters are quite concerned about tides, you can learn more about them by enrolling in a basic boating class at your local U.S. Coast Guard Auxiliary or U.S. Power Squadron.

Predicting the tidal current associated with tidal movement is also of value to a diver.

TIDAL CURRENTS

The tidal current is the horizontal flow of water caused by the tides. As shown in Fig. 12-2, when the flow is toward land, it is called flood current. When the flow is away from land it is called ebb current (Fig. 12-3). As the current changes direction, there is a time when no horizontal movement occurs. This point is referred to as the slack time, or slack water.

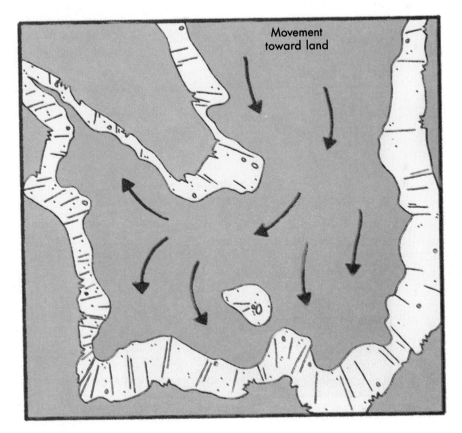

Movement toward land

Fig. 12-2 *Flood current.*

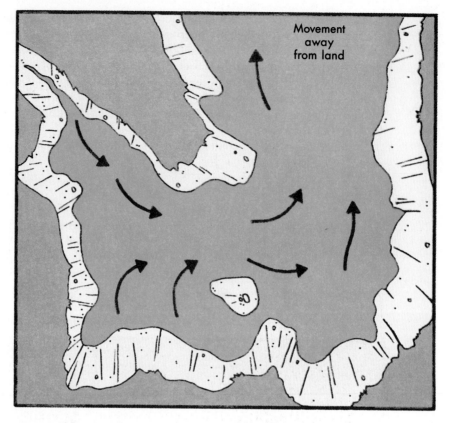

Movement
away
from land

Fig. 12-3 Ebb current.

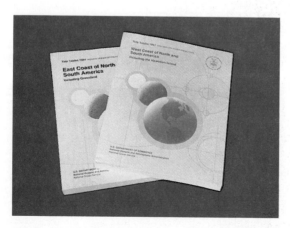

Fig. 12-4 Tidal Current Tables.

Tidal Current Tables

The times and speeds of tidal currents have been measured over many years at numerous coastal locations. As a result of these studies, a set of four tables has been developed by the National Ocean Service (NOS) to predict the current speed and direction at various locations, called reference and subordinate stations. Two books are published, one for the Pacific Coast of North America and Asia, and another for the Atlantic Coast (Fig. 12-4).

It is from these books that a diver can obtain time and speed of tidal currents for planning. A prudent diver certainly would not want to be swept out to sea by a strong ebb current unknowingly.

Even if all you have are Tide Tables, you can roughly predict the time of maximum current as half-way between a high and a low tide, but you will not be able to predict its speed.

OCEAN CURRENTS

Water movement occurring on a global scale is that created by ocean currents. Ocean currents are caused primarily by the sun's uneven heating of the earth's surface, the wind, and the rotation of the earth.

The sun heats equatorial waters faster than polar waters. As polar water freezes, the salt is squeezed out of the ice and falls into the unfrozen water. This cold, salty water is much heavier and denser so that it sinks into the depths, pushing the warmer water up and out of the way. The warmer water tends to rise up toward the earth's poles and the water is constantly warmed near the equator and cooled as it returns to the poles. Unceasing ocean currents thus occur all over the planet.

The uneven heating, together with worldwide wind patterns and the east-to-west rotation of the earth, creates six major circular currents in the oceans. One is in each hemisphere of the Pacific, Atlantic, and Indian Oceans. Currents in the northern hemisphere circulate in a clockwise direction, while those in the southern hemisphere travel in a counterclockwise direction.

WAVES

Waves form in essentially two ways: they are generated either by wind or by some geologic disturbance beneath the water (submarine earthquakes or volcanic eruptions).

Wind Waves

Wind waves are always born in the same way, whether it happens in the middle of the ocean or on the surface of a small pond. First the wind disturbs the surface of the water, as shown in Fig. 12-5. When the surface is disturbed, ripples appear. These ripples are actually caused by changes in air pressure on the surface and the frictional drag of the moving air. The ripples, though small, resist the wind. The wind pushes against the ripples until they become small waves.

Three factors determine how large a wave will become: how hard the wind blows (velocity); how long the wind blows (time); and over what distance the wind

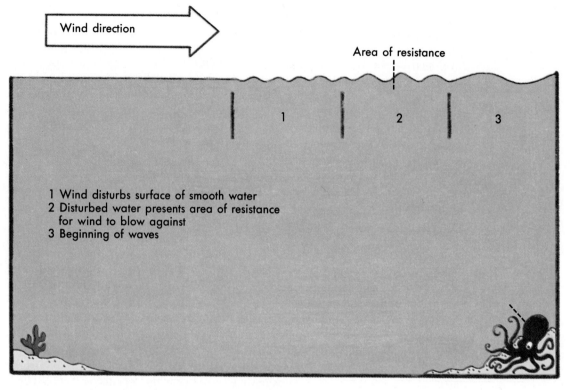

Wind direction

Area of resistance

1

2

3

1 Wind disturbs surface of smooth water
2 Disturbed water presents area of resistance
  for wind to blow against
3 Beginning of waves

Fig. 12-5 *Wave formation.*

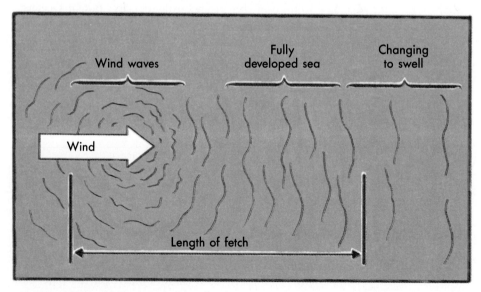

Wind waves

Fully
developed sea

Changing
to swell

Wind

Length of fetch

Fig. 12-6 *Waves, fetch, and swell.*

continues to blow (fetch) (Fig. 12-6). The harder the wind blows, the more quickly it disturbs the water. The newly formed wave presents a larger surface for the wind to blow against, and the result is an even larger wave. The longer and harder the wind blows, the larger the wave becomes.

If the wind remains constant, the water surface reaches a steady-state wave condition known as sea. Sea persists only as long as the wind keeps blowing and exists only in the fetch area. Swell waves (better known as swell) develop when the wind velocity decreases or the waves leave the fetch area (see Fig. 12-6). Swell waves have rounded crests and are longer than sea waves.

Because the wind pushes the water for a short distance, the water in a given wave appears to move. But it is actually the wave energy which is moving. The water rises and falls, as shown in Fig. 12-7. This principle can be illustrated with a length of rope. If you hold one end of a rope extended outward in a straight line along the ground and flip the rope several times, it will send a series of waves along the rope. The rope remains in the same place; only the energy moves to the other end. The energy from waves can travel almost indefinitely if unobstructed.

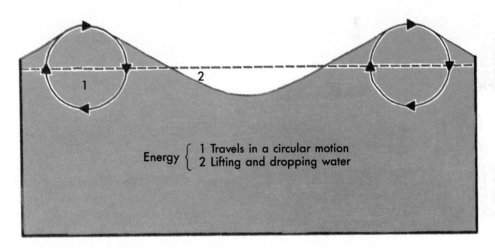

Energy { 1 Travels in a circular motion
         2 Lifting and dropping water

Fig. 12-7 *Energy motion in waves.*

Waves may grow to enormous proportions, often reaching 40 feet or more in height if the wind blows long and strong enough. The height of a wave, as shown in Fig. 12-8, is measured from the trough to the crest. The length is measured from crest to crest.

Formation of Surf

The waves created by offshore storms may eventually flatten to the point where they are no longer visible. But the energy is still moving. As the waves approach shallower water near the shore, the motion of the water particles beneath the surface is altered. The wave is said to "feel bottom" when it enters water of depth

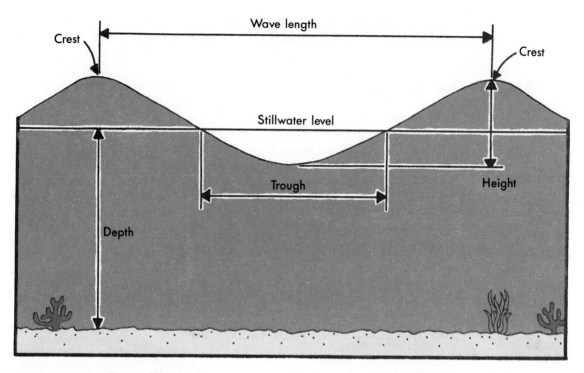

Fig. 12-8 *Wave measurements.*

equal to or less than one-half the wavelength. This makes the wave steeper and shorter.

As the wave height increases, the water particles at the crest orbit with increasing velocity. Finally, the wave breaks at approximately 1.3 times the wave height, when the steepest surface of the wave inclines more than 60° from the horizontal. These breaking waves (breakers) make up what is called the surf. The surf zone extends from where the waves first feel the bottom to just beyond the area of "white water," or where they have spent their energy.

Waves breaking away from the shore generally indicate a submerged reef or sandbar. Waves also break away from shore when they grow in height and steepness and the tops of the waves are blown off by strong winds. The crests of the waves fall under the force of gravity, causing broken water or white caps.

The primary problem for divers entering or exiting through surf is the weight of large quantities of water tumbling from the top of the wave to the shore. There can be tons of water in the breaking crest of large waves.

After the wave breaks, its water rushes up onto the beach face in what is called uprush. Once the water has rushed up onto the beach, it must return to the sea. This seaward movement of water is called backrush. This is often confused with the mythical undertow—a current said to flow seaward along the bottom and to pull swimmers under. Backrush may seem to pull a swimmer or diver under because it will pull the person toward the sea if he has been knocked down into it by another onrushing wave.

Sand Beach Entries

It is best to consult local divers concerning surf and bottom conditions before diving through surf on an unfamiliar beach. Since wave height and bottom configuration are directly related to surf conditions, you can obtain information on the height of the sea from wind data and on bottom configuration from the nautical chart, if no local divers are available.

The best information comes first-hand from actually watching the "beat" of the surf. Depending on how far offshore the waves were created, they will tend to stabilize into sets. A set of waves is the number of waves of various sizes which tends to repeat itself. Every once in a while, however, there may be a particularly large set of waves. Shore entries and exits should be timed to coincide with the smaller waves in a set.

The type of breakers rolling into shore also affects the method of entering through surf. When one breaks slowly over quite a distance, it is a spilling breaker (Fig. 12-9). A plunging breaker, as shown in Fig. 12-10, curls over and breaks in one big crash. A surging breaker does not spill or plunge, but peaks (Fig. 12-11). The steepness of the beach determines the type of breaker. There is a greater tendency for breakers to plunge or surge when the beach slope is steep.

After observing the surf beat and breaker patterns for a short time, you will know when to move into the water. Here is a procedure for entering the water through surf:

1. Have your mask and fins on and your regulator in your mouth. In some calm areas, fins are not put on until you are in about waist deep water. In dressing beforehand, be aware that any gear placed near the water's edge can be carried away easily by a large wave.
2. Hold onto your mask and regulator firmly to keep them in place, especially when breakers hit.
3. Slide or shuffle backward into the water rather than walking, to keep your balance better and avoid being surprised by stepping into a hole. Keeping your knees bent slightly helps with balance. When a wave hits you in shallow water move with it slightly to avoid being smacked by it.
4. When you are deep enough to swim, turn around and swim out through the surf with your regulator in your mouth. The surf disturbs a great deal of sand; your regulator may be filled with sand if it hangs loose.
5. Pass through the surf as quickly as possible. Make any equipment adjustments either after you pass through the surf zone or before, but definitely not in the surf.
6. The power of a wave is concentrated in the surface area. To avoid fighting that power, simply swim through or under the wave, not over it. Swim as low as possible, next to the bottom, to let the backrush help you.

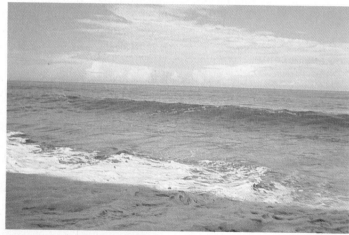

Fig. 12-9 Spilling breaker.

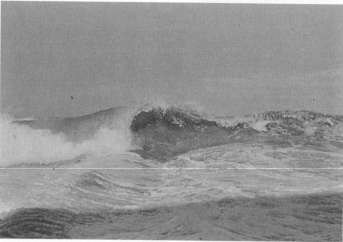

Fig. 12-10 Plunging breaker.

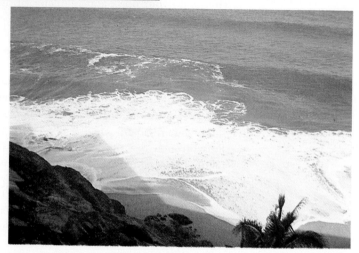

Fig. 12-11 Surging breaker.

Once you are past the surf zone, you and your buddy should rejoin and rest by inflating your buoyancy compensators before proceeding. Any extra items to be carried should be tied to a float and pulled through the surf rather than pushed. You should push the float when you return to shore, so the float will not be slammed into you by a wave.

Returning to shore is easier than entering. Just outside the surf zone you should stop, rest, observe the waves, and prepare to exit. Time your exit to swim in with the smaller breakers. Once you can touch bottom, do not stand up, but swim with the water as far up on shore as possible. Keep your regulator in your mouth as you did on entry to keep it clear of sand. Kneel when you can, and relax. Then crawl out of the water until you can stand without hazard. Take your fins off or shuffle backward until you are on dry ground.

A more complete discussion of beach diving is found in the *Advanced Manual*.

Freshwater Entries

Freshwater entries are essentially the same as for the ocean.

Rocky Shore Entries

A rocky entry is hazardous in that falling or being knocked down on rocks can cause injuries. To avoid possible injury, look for the least obstructed entry path and begin swimming as soon as possible, rather than walking on a rocky surface.

You can do this by being fully ready to go, then lying face down in the backrush of the last large wave of a set. Let this backrush carry you past the rocks by swimming in a prone position while facing the next wave. So you will not be pulled back onto shore by the next wave, hold onto a rock and kick, and continue on out to sea with the next backrush.

Exit on the back side of the last large wave in a set. Again, grasp a rock to avoid being carried out to sea with the backrush, then swim with the next uprush to go well up onto shore. Be extremely cautious when crawling over slippery rocks.

Coral Reef Entries

Entries around coral reefs should be made when there is sufficient water over the reef to let you swim over it. Since reefs are delicate and pocked with holes, a diver should never walk directly on the corals, to avoid both crushing the corals to death and cutting his or her feet. Instead, the entry is best made by walking or swimming through sand channels among the corals. Follow these channels through the reef into deep water. If no suitable passages are present in the immediate area, move along the reef until you find a good entry and exit area.

Surge

In deep water, wave action has little effect on the horizontal water movement. Therefore, a boat will move up and down with wave action, but it generally stays the same distance from shore. As a wave reaches more shallow water, the circular motion flattens to a back-and-forth movement due to the influence of the bottom. This back-and-forth movement is called surge. Surge is a nuisance to underwater photographers and collectors and can be dangerous in rocky areas, because its back-

and-forth movement prevents you from staying in one place, and it can bump you against rocks and other obstructions.

LOCALIZED CURRENTS

Longshore and rips are two types of currents present in and near the surf zone. They are generated when waves approach the shoreline at an angle, or by an irregular configuration of the bottom. They normally involve only the top few feet of water, and then only for a relatively short distance.

Longshore Currents

Longshore currents flow parallel to a beach and are generated from waves approaching the shore at an angle. You find them most frequently along straight beaches. Their speed seldom exceeds 1 knot, but it does increase with the height of the breakers, decreasing wave period, increasing breaker line angle with the beach, and increasing slope of the beach. A longshore current can easily carry you away from your entry/exit point.

Rip Currents

Rip currents flow out from the beach side of a surf zone usually. They are generated by a build-up of extra water put on the beach by a current or surf. A rip current

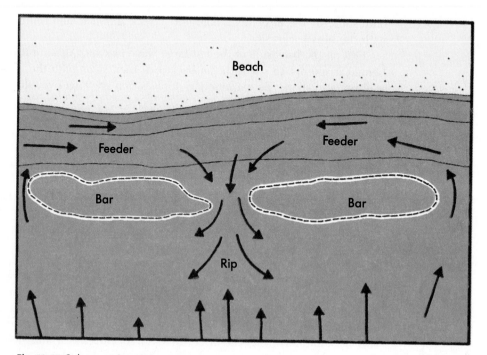

Fig. 12-12 *Submerged reef rip current.*

does nothing more than take the extra water back out into the ocean by the path of least resistance.

The easiest rip current to see is a stationary one created by two submerged bars or reefs as in Fig. 12-12. Surf carries water over the bars to the beach while the bars prevent its return to the ocean in backrush. The trapped water flows along the beach looking for an easy way out. In this case, the space between the bars lets the trapped water flow back to the ocean in a relatively high speed current. Even very strong swimmers are only able to maintain a maximum pace of less than 1 mph; swimming against a rip current, which can range from 3 to 12 mph, is a losing battle. It makes better sense to swim out of a rip current to its side if you are trying to get to shore. It also makes good sense to use the rip current as a fast transport out past the bar if you are going out to sea.

Along a long straight beach, as shown in Fig. 12-13, rip currents may appear in several places when the surf is strong enough to pile extra water up on the beach. The trapped water again travels along the beach looking for an easy way out. With no bars or reefs to help, slight depressions in the beaches act as conduits for rip currents, which is why there may be several close by.

Sometimes other currents cause rips, such as in Fig. 12-14. Part of the current is split off by the point, circles around, and meets head on with another part of the longshore current. The build-up of water has to move away from the beach, and it

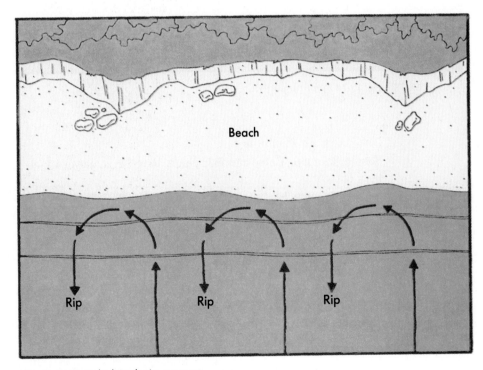

Fig. 12-13 *Straight beach rip currents.*

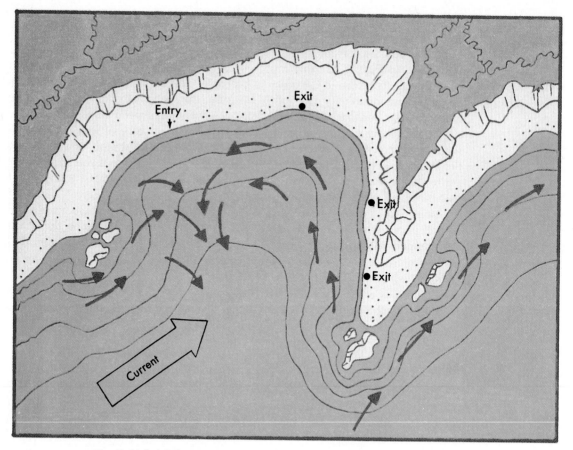

Fig. 12-14 *Point rip current.*

does so in a rip. Entry and exit points have been shown which take advantage of both currents.

Rip currents are recognized by two main characteristics: (1) the current is usually a different color than the surrounding water, and (2) the incoming surf height is lessened by the outgoing rip. To locate a rip, then, find a relatively narrow band of discolored water moving away from the beach where the surf is a bit reduced.

Effects of Currents on Boat Divers

Longshore currents are readily apparent when you dive from a boat, if you recognize their signs. One is that an anchored boat tends to swing into the current, as illustrated in Fig. 12-15. Another indication is via what you see floating by on the surface (including debris, seaweed, other divers, and the like).

Before entering the water, the diver should estimate the current's speed. If the current is much greater than 1 knot, dive some place else; if it is 1 knot or less, or a

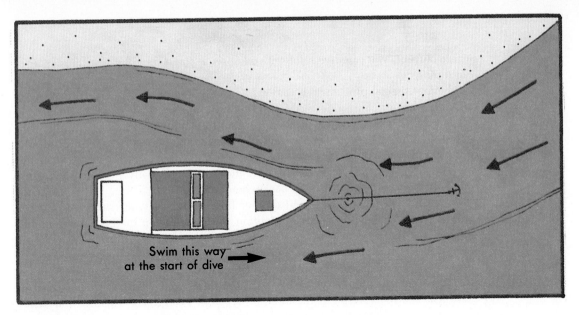

Fig. 12-15 *Current action near shore.*

Swim this way
at the start of dive

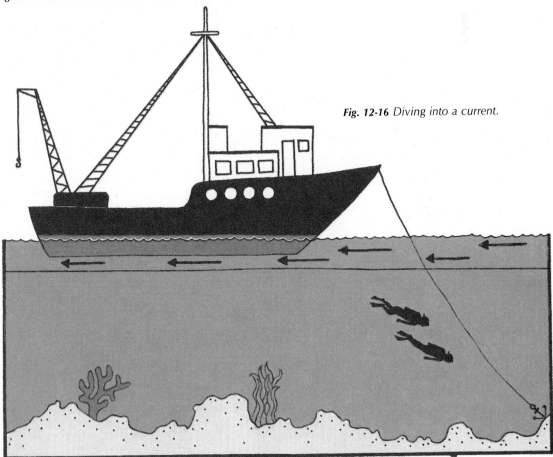

Fig. 12-16 *Diving into a current.*

surface current, you can dive safely, if you observe some special procedures for current diving.

The first special procedure is to descend to the bottom in a current either down the anchor line or along a descent line. That way, you will know what the current is on the bottom before you let go of the boat. You should always swim into the current at the beginning of a dive, as shown in Fig. 12-16. If you have to pull yourself over the rocks ahead of the boat, the current is too strong to dive safely and the dive should be aborted. It would be poor judgment to initially swim downcurrent, then fight the current on the way back when you are tired.

If you are carried downcurrent of your boat, be ready with certain safety precautions. Carry a whistle to attract attention of the people on the boat; the sound of a whistle carries farther than the voice on the windy surface, with much less effort. Always wear a buoyancy compensator that fits properly and is well maintained so you can rest for long periods of time on the surface.

The best divers are always prepared for the unexpected. Lack of preparation can cause fear and its resulting panic in a downcurrent emergency. Ensure your safety under any condition with preparation, proper equipment, and training. For a complete discussion of boat diving, consult the *Advanced Manual*.

13

Ocean Life

- Reefs
- Reef Inhabitants
- Dangerous Marine Animals
- Handling Marine Life

OBJECTIVES

At the conclusion of Chapter 13, you will be able to:

1. Name the two types of corals.
2. State two functions the coral reefs provide to the ecosystem.
3. Explain the formation of the three major reef structures.
4. Name the large algae found attached to rocks in colder water.
5. Describe how to perform the kelp crawl.
6. Explain normal barracuda behavior toward the scuba diver.
7. State how the diver can prevent moray eel bites.
8. Explain how to prevent sting ray injury in shallow water.
9. Name the type of injury received from fire coral.
10. State the best policy to follow in handling marine life.

KEY TERMS

Cnidaria	Scleractinia	Octocorallia
Symbiotic	Polyps	Porifera
Kelp	Anemone	Crustaceans
Biomass	Hydrozoa	

The ocean depths are a sightseer's dream. Their panorama is so vast that quite often the inexperienced diver sees very little of it. Life dwells on every rock and reef and in sand, and unless you familiarize yourself with these life forms, you might miss the most enjoyable part of the dive.

Another thing to consider is that despite their beauty and fascination, some creatures present potential hazards. The diver who studies the new surroundings underwater can appreciate and understand them well enough to avoid personal harm during all underwater excursions.

Underwater animals have one thing in common with their untamed relatives on land—they are wild. Most water creatures are neither aggressive nor friendly. They are often indifferent to strange invaders to their domain. While some may be a little curious, most become cautious when they see a diver, and you should remember that some are capable of inflicting serious injury when molested. Most injury, however, is the result of the sea creature reacting to disturbance rather than from aggression. Because some wounds can be serious, it is wise to know exactly which animals you can touch, and which ones to avoid.

REEF DEVELOPMENT

Corals

Corals are members of the phylum Cnidaria. They are found in both hard and soft forms and are related to hydroids, hydras, jellyfishes, and sea anemones. The hard

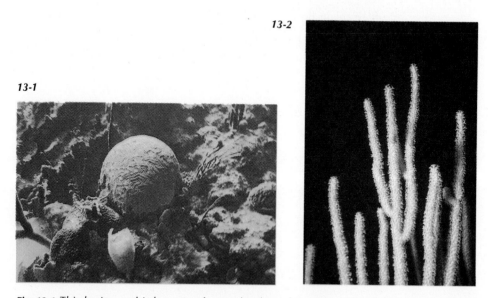

13-1

13-2

Fig. 13-1 *This brain coral is but one of many hard corals you may see diving among tropical and subtropical reefs.*

Fig. 13-2 *Looking more like what we have come to recognize as a plant, this is one of the soft corals which is in fact colonies of many thousands of the separate anthozoans.*

corals (Fig. 13-1) (Scleractinia) resemble rocks, while soft corals (Octocorallia) resemble plants (Fig. 13-2). Both are large contributors to reef formation.

Corals reproduce both sexually by interacting with other corals, and asexually by dividing. The way in which they reproduce determines the formation of coral. New colonies develop when the coral reproduces sexually by releasing eggs and sperm, which unite, then float along with the current to new places. There they settle to the bottom in shallow water and attach themselves to anything solid. Older colonies grow when coral reproduces by dividing, to add more members to the colonies.

Due to several factors, including temperature, water movement, sunlight, and the availability of solid objects, coral is limited to the relatively shallow depths in warm waters. Some are too delicate to survive in areas of violent water action. Others grow right up to the low tide level and even protrude slightly out of the water.

Corals provide shelter to reef inhabitants. They also provide a symbiotic home for zooxanthella, an alga which lives in and makes oxygen for coral polyps (Fig. 13-3), which in turn supply carbon dioxide for the alga. This alga gives color to most corals and furnishes the chemistry for the actual formation of the coral structure.

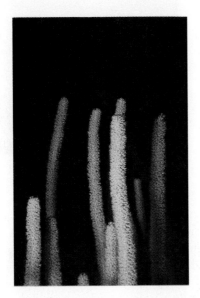

Fig. 13-3 *This closeup of a pillar coral shows the detail of the individual polyps that make up the coral colony.*

Corals are a source of food for many creatures that eat the coral and leave a residue of sand. Corals are a significant part, if not the entire basis, for the ecosystem in warm waters, where coral reefs provide shelter, food, and protection from their inhabitants' enemies. It is difficult to conceive of oceans without coral reefs.

Corals may also be fragile organisms that can be killed by the rough touch of a diver's glove, the strong kick of a fin, the hard contact with a tank, or the fall of a boat's anchor. It is prudent then that divers do all they can to limit their contact with coral and when necessary touch it gently, be aware of possible fin contact situations, maintain neutral buoyancy, and set the boat anchors nondestructively in clear areas to preserve living corals for future diving excursions.

Corals of all kinds are extremely fragile organisms, and simply touching living coral tends to kill or shorten the life expectancy of virtually thousands of organisms. Therefore, it is important that divers do all they can to maintain neutral buoyancy, watch what their fins contact, keep their equipment tight to their bodies so it does not touch living things, and avoid touching all marine organisms that may be delicate.

Sponges

Another large contributor to reef building is the sponge (Porifera)—an animal, not a plant. Sponges come in every size, shape, color, and texture (Fig. 13-4). Though not edible by humans, their skeletons, in which the actual animal lives, are used by humans for cleaning and other household chores.

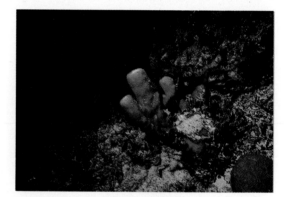

Fig. 13-4 The tube sponge is an example of the many varieties of sponges that you may see while diving.

Reef Formation and Depths

Three distinct reef formations are illustrated in Fig. 13-5: the deep reef found at 80 to 100 feet deep; the midreef found in the 20- to 40-foot range; and the shallow reef found from 15 feet up to sea level. These have been formed during recent geological eras when the prevailing seas have been at different sea levels.

It appears that the surfaces of the oceans were once near the level of the deep reef. The midreef formed as the waters rose. We are now seeing the development of the shallow reef with the water at its present level.

Small individual clumps of one or more coral animal colonies grow in the shallow reef. In the midreef areas, corals have had time to grow together and form larger overlapping clumps. These look like small islands; many are as large as 50 to 75 feet, but they remain as separate and distinct coral clumps. In the deep reef, the clumps or small islands have had an opportunity to grow together, forming one continuous reef cut intermittently by ravines, and large and small caves created partly by worms, which eat into the coral and weaken it, causing breakage. The reefs also become honeycombed because the various corals grow and overlap each other.

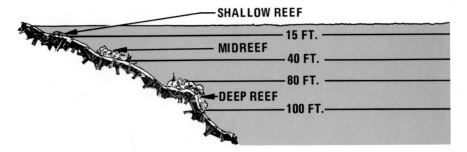

Fig. 13-5 *The various reef levels that have been formed in the world's tropical and subtropical oceans.*

Though a reef may appear to be like solid rock, it is a network of caves and passageways.

Water temperature also limits the area in which coral can flourish. Since most coral requires temperatures above 75° F (24° C), it is restricted to the band of ocean waters between 30 degrees north and 30 degrees south of the equator. Interestingly enough, coral reefs are found only on the eastern shores of the continents. This is probably due to the cold water currents on the western side of the continents.

Bottom Formation in Cold Waters

In cold water areas which lack the warmth to produce hard corals, bottom formations are composed primarily of rock. In some areas, the coastline is lined with kelp beds.

Rocks and kelp provide the same kind of protection for sea animals in cold water regions that coral provides in warmer waters. While cold waters normally do not produce the profusion of different individual animals that warm waters do, the population in terms of numbers of animals in cold water is more extensive, especially in the kelp forests.

Kelp, an alga, attaches itself to rocks with a holdfast in as much as 50 to 75 feet of water. Its stipes (stalks) grow from the bottom to the surface, sometimes as fast as 2 feet per day. Kelp fronds (leaves) are normally several feet apart, but when they reach the surface, they lay in a mat. A kelp bed resembles a forest with the leaf-covered branches of the trees intertwining and shutting out the sun in many places. Kelp is a wonderful place to dive because it contains more sea life than one might imagine possible (Fig. 13-6).

There have been frightening stories of divers becoming entangled in kelp. Underwater, you can avoid entanglement just by watching where you are going. On the surface, a diver who remains calm can use a kelp crawl to move over a kelp bed with relative ease. To move across kelp, push it down very slowly with your forearm and hand, then pull your floating body over it. Let your fins just drag behind, not kicking. Move slowly and methodically, forcing the kelp down with your arms. If you do become entangled, kelp can be broken, cut, or removed with the help of your buddy, a reasonably sharp knife.

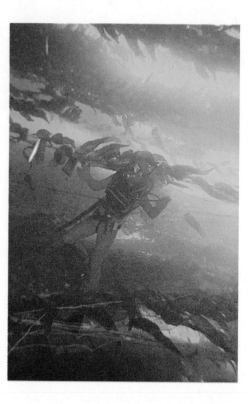

Fig. 13-6 Diving in the kelp on the United States' west coast.

REEF INHABITANTS

The reef makeup, whether coral or rock, is extremely complex. Its biomass (life forms) ranges from the smallest microorganism in coral to sponges, shellfish, crustaceans, fish, and even plants. Large free-swimming pelagic fish, which use the reef as a source of food and as a breeding area, may also be part of the reef's ecosystem. Each animal serves its special function within this underwater environment.

By watching a reef for a period of time, you can start to figure out the existing territorial system. A big fish may preside over an entire section of a large reef as a reef master. Under its control, the reef is divided into territories. The size of the territory depends upon the size of the fish, extending down to the smallest fish that may inhabit no more than a few cubic inches.

To the new diver, the most apparent reef inhabitants are fish. Some typical tropical fish are described below.

The parrotfish, as seen in Fig. 13-7, is one of the most active members of the reef community. They eat the living coral animals by biting off pieces of the coral structure to get at the animal. In so doing, they grind it up, making sand, with the adult parrotfish producing about 1 acre of sand yearly. They also eat algae which help keep coral healthy. In terms of collective pounds, they make up the biggest weight of reef inhabitants.

Porgies of different types have a similar appearance, differing mostly in color. They weigh, in adulthood, between 2 and 4 pounds and are found throughout the

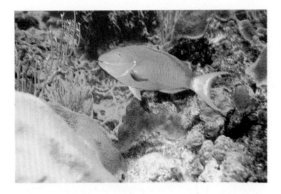

Fig. 13-7 The stoplight parrotfish.

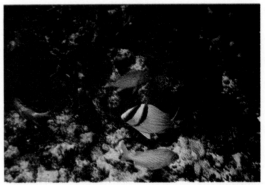

Fig. 13-8 Porkfish are the prettiest example of the porgy.

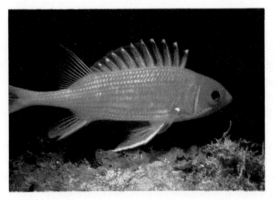

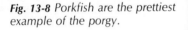

Fig. 13-9 Squirrel fish.

tropics. The most outstanding example of the porgy is the blue, yellow, and black porkfish, shown in Fig. 13-8.

The squirrel fish is aptly named. Its big brown eyes give it almost a comic look, as seen in Fig. 13-9.

Angel fish are among the most beautiful on the reef and appear quite graceful. The French angel, shown in Fig. 13-10, is black with scales outlined in yellow. This fish almost glows in its brilliance. A cousin, the gray angel, shown in Fig. 13-11, has almost no fear of man and can be touched occasionally. The queen angel, shown in

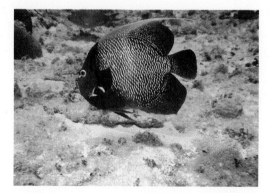

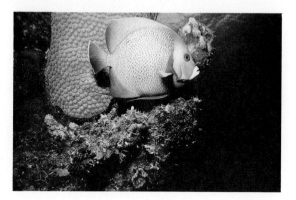

Fig. 13-10 French angel.

Fig. 13-11 Gray angel.

Fig. 13-12, is considered by some as the most beautiful of the angel fish. Its brilliant colors change with each shift of light.

Invertebrates

Fish are often the ocean inhabitants the diver sees first, but they comprise only a small part of the total population. Another common inhabitant on sand or reef is the starfish. The starfish, shown in Fig. 13-13, is one of the bottom dwellers that will be found clinging to rocks or crawling across the bottom. The main food of the starfish is shellfish and barnacles. Starfishes may have as few as four arms but, in the case of the feather star, may have up to 20 arms. The starfish skeleton is a loose meshwork of calcareous plates or rods.

The sea urchin, a variety of which are shown in Fig. 13-14, is found in oceans throughout the world. It is nature's pincushion, because it has needle-like spines that protrude from its body in all directions. Its body is a small globular shell usually seen only after the sea urchin's death when the spines have fallen off.

The sea anemone is a marine animal that looks like a plant and is in the same phylum as coral, jellyfish, and hydroids. Anemones range in size from a fraction of an inch to over 1 foot in diameter. Many look like flowers, as shown in Fig. 13-15. Their tentacles contain nematocysts (stinging cells) which inject toxic substances into their prey.

Featherduster worms, shown in Fig. 13-16, are further evidence of the overlap in appearance between plant and animal. The dusters' flowerlike plumage is actually used to breathe and attract food. They are less than 8 inches high and many are barely visible. They are found on the bottom in sand or growing in coral, and appear to be more plentiful in shallow water. As you might imagine, they are quite fragile and retract at the slightest touch. Another example is the spiral Christmas tree worm, shown in Fig. 13-17.

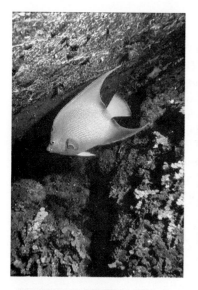

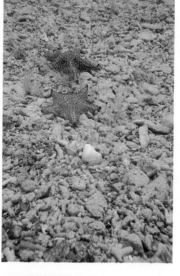

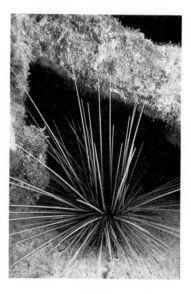

13-12

13-13

13-14

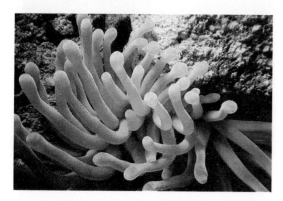

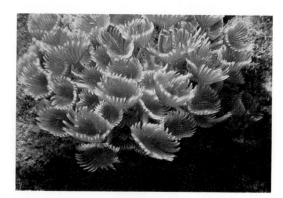

13-15

13-16

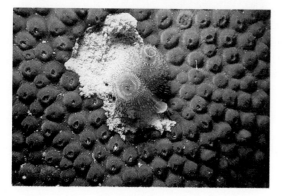

Fig. 13-12 Queen angel.

Fig. 13-13 Starfish.

Fig. 13-14 The long-spined sea urchin.

Fig. 13-15 Closeup photo of the tentacles of the strawberry anemone.

Fig. 13-16 Featherduster worms.

Fig. 13-17 Christmas tree worm.

13-17

Crustaceans

Careful observation in the little nooks and crannies of a reef will expose many creatures like the banded coral shrimp pictured in Fig. 13-18. This tiny coral shrimp is only about 1 inch long and is nearly transparent. They are primarily nocturnal and their transparency helps protect them from enemies.

The arrow shrimp, like the banded coral shrimp, is somewhat shy during the day. It may be found walking among coral reefs, cleaning up bits and pieces of debris that make up its diet. Like many of the crustaceans, the arrow crab, pictured in Fig. 13-19, is one of the ocean's "cleaner uppers."

The spiny lobster, shown in Fig. 13-20, is a popular food source for divers in tropical waters. It differs from the clawed lobster, in that it has no large front claws but has a longer tail relative to body length. Lobsters grow to over 20 pounds, although 12 pounds is considered large.

Fig. 13-18 *Banded coral shrimp.*

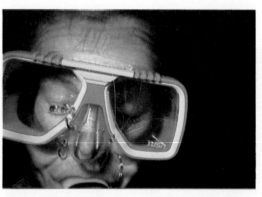

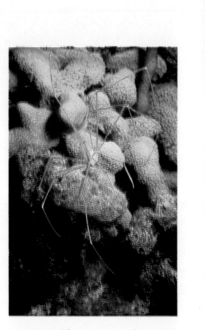

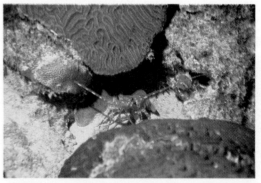

Fig. 13-19 *The arrow crab, another of the reef's small crustacean inhabitants.*

Fig. 13-20 *The spiny lobster.*

DANGEROUS MARINE ANIMALS

For the most part, animals that present a risk to the scuba diver are local or regional in nature and you can best learn about those creatures that present a risk to you from the divers in the area where you are planning your dive. However, there are a few ocean environs that deserve special mention.

The shark has been greatly overstated as a risk to the scuba diver. Since the release of the book and movie "Jaws," many people who frequent the ocean are looking around every corner for the next man-eating great white shark.

Though there are 350 species of shark identified worldwide, only about 25 species have ever been connected with attacks on humans. The few attacks that have involved scuba divers have also usually involved dead or wounded fish being carried by the divers back from a hunt in an area known to be frequented by sharks. To diminish the risk of shark attack, do not carry bait or dead fish around underwater.

Since most scuba divers never have an opportunity to see shark up close, it can be the highlight of a dive (Fig. 13-21). Sharks are large creatures which can swim gracefully and very fast. They are one of nature's scavengers assigned to keeping the ocean clear of dead and dying animals. Most sharks view the scuba diver, a rather large animal too, as a threat and retreat before the diver ever sees them. If a shark is encountered on a dive, and you feel uncomfortable about being there, simply leave the area with as little commotion as possible. Stay underwater, on the bottom if possible, and keep your eyes on the shark to see its reaction to your leaving. When the opportunity presents itself, exit the water and share your shark encounter with your dive buddies in words.

The barracuda, like the shark, is an overrated threat to divers (Fig. 13-22). Though they look vicious with their open mouths full of teeth, these fish have yet to be accused of an unbaited attack. Usually, their habit is to approach a diver slowly

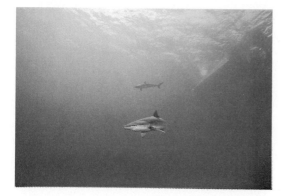

Fig. 13-21 Seeing a shark on a dive can be a thrilling experience, and most divers have not had the opportunity to view one up close.

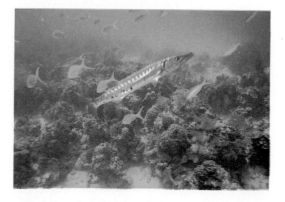

Fig. 13-22 Another overrated threat to the diver is the barracuda, a friendly and rather intelligent ocean dweller.

to within about 4 feet, but no closer, then just hang around. Unless you expose some food (bait), a barracuda may be just another dive buddy.

The moray eel is another of the oceans' creatures which prefers to avoid divers, is shy in nature, and usually nocturnal in behavior (Fig. 13-23). The bite of a moray can be very nasty and is easily avoided by not putting your hands into holes and crevices while diving. If you put your hand into a hole where an eel lives, the creature feels threatened and will defensively bite to protect itself and its territory.

The sting ray, a variety of which is shown in Fig. 13-24, does not sting as its name implies. The threat this creature presents is a spine at the base of its tail. Injuries from this fish usually occur when someone wading in shallow water steps on one buried in the sand. Other injuries sometimes occur on the deck of a fishing

13-23

13-24

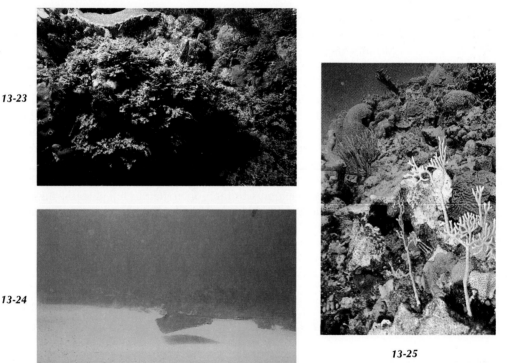

13-25

Fig. 13-23 *The moray eel is usually seen on night dives but may sometimes be seen by the observant diver during the day. Avoiding injury from the moray eel is simply a matter of keeping your hands out of holes and crevices that you cannot visually inspect for other occupants.*

Fig. 13-24 *Caribbean sting ray. A graceful creature which really presents no threat to the diver who wades carefully in shallow water.*

Fig. 13-25 *Fire coral is definitely one of the "don't touch" creatures you will see while diving in tropical and subtropical waters.*

boat when a fisherman is struck by the spine of a flopping sting ray on the deck of the boat. For a diver, avoiding sting ray injuries is simply a matter of shuffling your feet as you enter the water where there is a sandy bottom and sting rays may be present.

Although in the same phylum as true corals, fire coral is actually a hydrozoa and not a true coral. These colonies, shown in Fig. 13-25, generally have a "melted" appearance and take many shapes varying from branching to platelike. The colors range from brown to creamy. The diver should avoid all contact with fire coral, since each of the pores in the colony contains polyps that produce a severe burning sensation and blistery rash following contact. A dive skin or light wet suit can protect the diver from accidental contact.

HANDLING MARINE LIFE

The best way to handle unfamiliar aquatic life is to not handle it at all. But if you must, do so with great care and gently to avoid injuring whatever living creature you encounter.

The defenses of marine life include size, speed, camouflage, barbs, stingers, and teeth. Most species that would seem to permit handling also have effective defense mechanisms.

As a general rule, therefore, look at, photograph, follow, but do not touch. Generally, you pose more of a threat to their existence than they do to yours. Adhering to this hands-off policy will keep you both out of trouble and protect and preserve the marine environment for all of us. As such, the greatest threat of injury will be caused by inadvertently and accidentally bumping into or stepping on something with spines, barbs, or sharp edges. The majority of serious diving accidents are the fault of the diver and not the marine environment.

SUMMARY

Ocean life continues to be fascinating and sometimes mysterious to those who seek to unlock its endless array of secrets. By constantly learning more about the oceans, we will be able to enjoy and use them to benefit them, their inhabitants, and us.

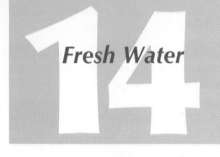

Fresh Water

- Lakes
- Rivers
- Sandpits and Quarries
- Natural Caves and Caverns
- Sinkholes and Springs
- Mines
- Animal Life

OBJECTIVES

At the conclusion of Chapter 14, you will be able to:

1. Name at least five different fresh-water diving venues.

2. Describe two skills which might be needed to adapt the ocean diver for fresh-water diving.

3. Explain why a diver needs more or less weight in fresh water than in salt water.

4. State where 18 percent of the world's liquid fresh water is found.

5. Name one thing that might attract a diver to river diving.

6. Name the two organizations that could serve as references to a diver with an interest in cave diving.

7. Name the fish commonly referred to as the fresh-water barracuda.

8. Name the four types of amphibians found in fresh water.

9. Name the three classes of reptile that one might encounter while diving.

10. Name two mammals that might be seen while diving.

KEY TERMS

Sandpit	Quarry	Cave
Sinkhole	Overhead	Artifacts
Dredging	NACD	NSS-CDS

From the time recreational diving began, it has always been most closely associated with the oceans. There are, however, a significant number of divers who, either by choice or by circumstance, dive regularly in fresh water (Fig. 14-1). The ocean diver may find it difficult to imagine diving in a lake, quarry, or river but after shooting the rapids on scuba in a river, or exploring a steam shovel submerged in a quarry, or visiting a sunken town in a manmade lake, the ocean diver will probably find it much easier. Each type of diving environment has its own unique challenges and rewards, and with appropriate training, equipment, and preparation, a qualified diver can enjoy any dive site.

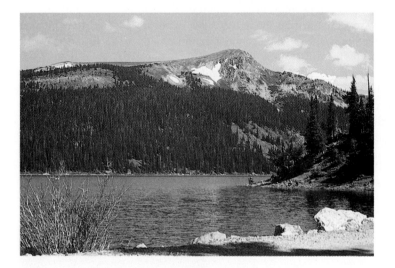

Fig. 14-1 *Scuba diving is not limited to the oceans but can be enjoyed equally well in fresh water.*

Diving Areas

Fresh water offers a great variety of locations for diving. There are lakes, rivers, sandpits, quarries, caves, sinkholes, springs, and even swamps. In fact, any place where there is water a few feet deep means possible diving to the avid diver.

Fresh water provides an array of interesting places to dive, and the exciting activities can be just as varied as any ocean dive site. Fresh-water dive sites offer the fortunate diver exciting opportunities for prospecting, collecting, and underwater photography.

Although the training is basically the same, fresh-water divers apply the skills differently in order to cope with potentially colder temperatures, limited visibility, and other potential hazards not regularly encountered by their ocean counterparts. Activities such as cave, cavern, under ice, and wreck diving (all called "overhead" environments) require significant amounts of additional training and a degree of capability not required of ocean divers. (See Chapter 18.)

While fresh water lacks the sea's variety of colorful and abundant life, still a wide assortment of fish and invertebrates thrive there. As with the ocean, every dive site—be it river, pond, or lake—deserves your attention and appreciation as a diver.

LAKES

Lakes are the largest venue for inland diving, ranging in size from a few acres to the Great Lakes, the huge fresh-water seas in the northern part of the United States. The Great Lakes, as a matter of fact, contain 18 percent of the world's liquid fresh water (Fig. 14-2).

Besides natural lakes, there are artificial lakes of every size in existence or being developed all over North America. These lakes or reservoirs are generally created by altering the natural flow of rivers. As the lakes form, a whole new ecosystem evolves. The diver exploring reservoirs can witness a chain of life that differs from that of natural lakes.

Because all structures which may present potential hazards to boating are removed, diving activities in new man-made lakes are generally limited to exploring and photography. New man-made lakes may not contain many artifacts and may not have established populations of aquatic life. They may, however, have new "treasures" in the form of lost boats, motors, and fishing tackle. Diving for these treasures is not only challenging, it is fun, and can also be financially rewarding.

Natural lakes, on the other hand, offer the greatest diving potential. They are normally clear and, depending upon their location, may be full of old relics. With the constant desire for memorabilia and antiques, there is hardly a better place to look than in natural lakes. The early settlers used the lakes and practically all bodies

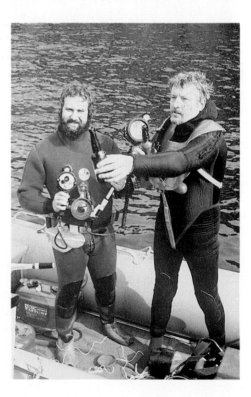

Fig. 14-2 The Great Lakes offer excellent diving and are the source of 18 percent of the world's fresh water.

of water as handy disposal areas. These areas can now be explored by sport divers who are looking for ways to combine their love of sport with an interest in history or antiques. Because fresh water does not affect metals as salt water does, most items can be salvaged in a very good state of preservation. It is advised, however, to become familiar with local and regional salvage laws so you can enjoy your sport without fear of breaking the law.

Wherever railroads were built over or near natural waters, artifacts abound. The railroaders had a habit of throwing trash, such as old bottles, into the water. You may also be able to find items lost during the construction of railroad bridges across lakes and rivers. It is rumored that more than one Colorado mountain lake contains gold and other valuable artifacts from old wrecked trains.

The Great Lakes are large enough to accommodate some of the largest steam and cargo vessels ever built. Ocean-going vessels have plied the waters of the Great Lakes since the late nineteenth century. Storms, collisions, and navigational mishaps have resulted in countless numbers of steel and wooden hull wrecks containing valuable and historically significant artifacts and treasure (Fig. 14-3).

RIVERS

River diving can be exciting (Fig. 14-4). Rivers, having been vitally important in early exploration, transportation, and commerce, contain artifacts chronicling the

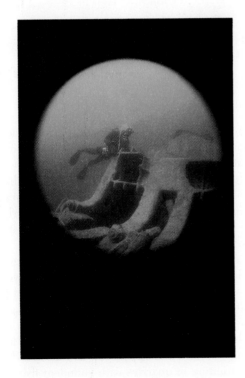

Fig. 14-3 *This is but one of countless wrecks found in the Great Lakes.*

early development of the country. No matter where you live in North America, you are probably not far from a river. While not all rivers are deep or clear enough to justify diving, many offer the qualified diver exciting potential. Underwater photography, artifact collecting, and gold dredging are just a few of the possibilities. For the adventuresome and dedicated diving enthusiast, gold dredging is an exciting and potentially rewarding hobby. Diving for gold, which is sometimes found in remote areas of Alaska, the Rocky Mountains, and California, requires a level of physical and financial commitment not found in other aspects of the sport.

Underwater photography, although potentially more challenging than in lakes, may offer the experienced river diver an opportunity for unusual photographs of aquatic life and shipwrecks not normally seen in other diving environments.

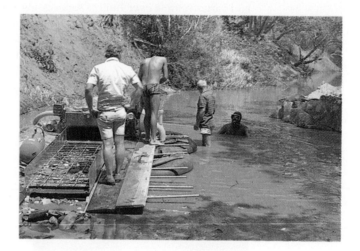

Fig. 14-4 *River diving.*

SANDPITS AND QUARRIES

A sandpit, gravel, or stone quarry is a small body of water, a few acres at best, artificially formed by removing natural mineral deposits. Actual stone quarries contain large pieces of mined stone, and the stone bottom is usually covered with a fine silt. Stone quarries are generally clear, and may be quite deep. The flooded stone quarry may contain structures left there once mining was abandoned. These structures may include steel-reinforced concrete structures that formerly housed rock-crushing machinery, huge scales for weighing tons of mined limestone, and other remnants of the once-active quarrying business.

Quarries may also contain objects specifically placed underwater for the interest and delight of the diver. School buses, automobiles, boats, and even aircraft have been placed in long-abandoned stone quarries to provide attractions for sport divers (Fig. 14-5). Since water enters an abandoned stone quarry as seepage from the surrounding groundwater, the visibility is generally quite good during most of the year. Gravel quarries, on the other hand, may contain large quantities of suspended clay particles, thus reducing visibility and appeal for diving. Spearfishing and general exploring can be quite exciting in quarries with abundant fish life.

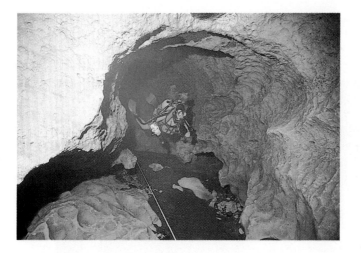

Fig. 14-5 *Quarry diving.*

Sandpits are formed when sand is removed from the existing spring area; the bottoms are normally sand, covered with a light layer of silt. Sandpits offer possibilities for photography, spearfishing, and occasional fossil hunting.

One thing that should be remembered about fresh-water lakes and rivers is that the land animals in the area depend on that water for sustenance. Because of the broad range of land animals, amphibians, and fish life that depend on the waters, nature can be observed at every level, much more readily than in the ocean. In fact, the observant diver can occasionally get a glimpse of a complete land/water ecosystem, particularly in arid regions where water is not abundant.

NATURAL CAVES

Natural caves are normally above water, and speleologists are the people who explore them. They occasionally run into water which, depending upon the cave's formation, may block an entrance to another part of the cave. It would seem appropriate for the dry-cave explorer to consider training in cave diving in order to continue exploration of such a system.

The vast majority of cave-diving activity is done in systems which have no such air-filled chambers or no known connections with dry caves (Fig. 14-6). Cave diving necessitates training and equipment far beyond that required of any other underwater activity. *No level of open-water training—including instructor—is sufficient to prepare divers to safely enter water-filled caves or caverns* (Fig. 14-7). For those interested in training and certification as cave divers, the following organizations represent the standard of cave diver training in the United States:

The National Association for Cave
   Diving (NACD)
P.O. Box 14492
Gainesville, FL 32604

The National Speleological Society—
   Cave Diving Section
(NSS-CDS)
P.O. Box 950
Branford, FL 32008

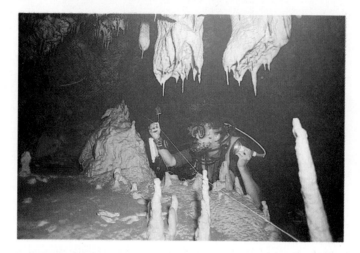

Fig. 14-6 Cave diving.

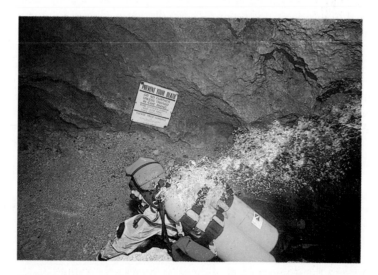

Fig. 14-7 A sign warning untrained divers NOT to cave dive.

SINKHOLES AND SPRINGS

Sinkholes and springs can be extremely deep and may actually lead into cave systems. Like all potential overhead environments, sinkholes and springs can be rather dangerous to dive in and may require a great amount of special training and equipment. Because of exceptional water clarity and relatively warm, constant water temperatures of around 72° F (23° C), they are very popular to visiting divers and offer excellent opportunities for photography. A number of sinkholes in Florida contain actual prehistoric animal bones and other remnants of the region's past, such as sharks' teeth. Artifacts which may have regional or national historical significance should be reported to local authorities. Certain states require permits to look for artifacts within state boundaries.

In some areas, like the mountains of Wyoming and Colorado, there are hot springs having high mineral content and extremely warm water, sometimes over 100° F (38° C).

MINES

Abandoned mines can provide exciting diving and are quite often very clear. Many contain relics, which make exploring and photography a natural activity. Because of high mineral content, there may be no animal life. Mines are normally deep and at the base of the open pit, there is often a mine shaft. Like diving in other overhead environments, this is not an open water diving adventure but may be an exciting dive for those trained and equipped to dive in specialized overhead environments.

COMMON FRESH-WATER ANIMALS

The fresh waters of North America, lack the immense variety of fish found in the oceans. Depending on the location and the water temperature, however, you can find a considerable variety of fresh-water aquatic life.

Fresh water, like salt water, contains a wide variety of fish of which some are edible, some not. In a few cases, the fish may be edible, but due to their eating habits or the water quality, are not desirable. Undesirable fish are referred to as nongame or trash fish. Whether or not a fish is a trash or a game fish depends partly on the area of the country. What is considered a trash fish in one place may be considered a game fish in another. This section is an introduction to a few of the fresh-water inhabitants a diver might encounter. There are many creatures which exist in the fresh-water environment that are very rarely, if ever, seen.

Fish

Small members of the sunfish family are found virtually all over North America (Fig. 14-8). They occasionally represent the majority of fish species in shallow-water lakes, ponds, rivers, and streams. Weighing up to 1 pound, they are prized by anglers, young and old alike. Like their distant ocean cousin, the damselfish, they exhibit territorial behavior and have been known to bite. Luckily, their small size precludes any real danger. Because of their curious nature, they make great subjects for underwater photographers.

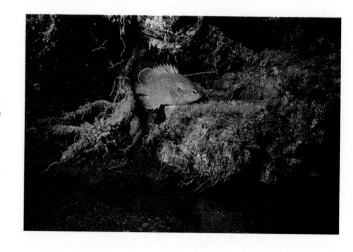

Fig. 14-8 The sunfish may also be known as a pumpkin seed, bream, or other local names.

The long streamlined northern pike is the most common fresh-water fish in the world. They are, however, most common in the northern United States and Canada. Because of their canine teeth and voracious appetite, they are sometimes called the fresh-water barracuda. Shy by nature, the northern pike, like all other large inhabitants of the fresh-water world, is seen by only a fortunate few.

Amphibians

Amphibians include frogs, toads, newts, and salamanders. Frogs and toads spend most or all of their life cycle in or near the water. They often provide a chirping or croaking chorus for night-diving enthusiasts yet are very rarely seen (Fig. 14-9). Ardent underwater photographers may have to inspect the extreme shallows to catch a glimpse of these amphibians, though approximately 70 different species are found in North America. Salamanders, with approximately 85 species in North America, are also often sought but rarely seen.

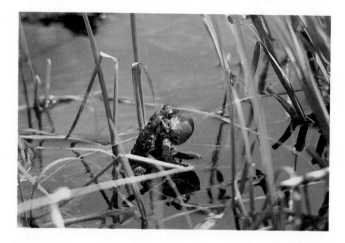

Fig. 14-9 A cautious diver/photographer, who carefully prowls the periphery of the fresh-water pond, may come upon a frog looking for a mate.

Reptiles

Three of the four major groups of reptiles found in North America are common in fresh-water rivers, lakes, and ponds—turtles, snakes, and alligators (Fig. 14-10). Alligators are the least common with the exception being in certain areas of the southeast (Fig. 14-11). Reptiles are major predators in the fresh-water food chain. All of these are capable of inflicting serious injury, even if only in a protective rather than aggressive response to a diver's presence.

Mammals

Fresh-water mammals are few, but the list does include manatees and beavers. Encounters with any one of these underwater creatures would definitely be worth writing about in your dive log. Of these, the manatee is the only nonhuman which may be viewed regularly by divers in fresh water. Manatees are quite common in the fresh waters of Florida, where they spend the winter months. These mammals are protected and have protected habitats. They are best viewed while skin diving because noise tends to keep them away. Efforts are currently underway to protect the manatee from extinction (Fig. 14-12). These creatures, like all inhabitants of the underwater world, deserve our understanding, appreciation, and protection.

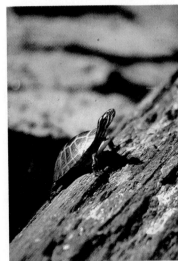

14-10

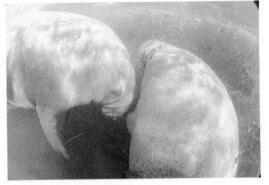

14-11

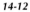

14-12

Fig. 14-10 *Being cold blooded, reptiles like this eastern painted turtle are often found on sunny days basking where they can get the maximum advantage of the warming rays of the sun.*

Fig. 14-11 *Alligators are best seen from a distance when diving, and the prudent diver avoids diving in areas known to be frequented by them.*

Fig. 14-12 *The manatee, the gentle "sea cow," which is seriously endangered.*

Ecology

15

- Sources of Problems
- Sewage and Garbage
- Construction

- Chemical Dumping
- Crude Oil Damage

- Commercial Fishing
- Sport Diving
- Inland Problems
- Solutions

OBJECTIVES

At the conclusion of Chapter 15, you will be able to:

1. Explain the significance of the chain of life.
2. Describe the meaning of a symbiotic relationship.
3. State the cause of certain marine life mutations.
4. Explain the environmental dangers that may be caused by dredging and land-fills near the water.
5. State the two major causes of oil spills.
6. Describe the impact on the ecosystem of today's commercial fishing.
7. Explain responsible spearfishing behavior for sport divers.
8. Tell the most significant diving behavior that will limit inadvertent environmental damage by sport divers.
9. Describe the environmental risk secondary to runoff.
10. Explain what resulting environmental damage is caused by acid rain.

KEY TERMS

Symbiosis	Mutations	Red tide
Estuaries	Aquifer	Pesticides
Herbicides	Eutrophication	Acid rain

SOURCES OF PROBLEMS

The balance of nature is really a wonderfully simple thing. In nature there is a chain of life wherein every living thing, be it plant or animal, provides either food or shelter for some other living thing (Fig. 15-1). Every creature, in order to live, must have food. If you somehow affect or remove its source of food, the creature suffers and may even die.

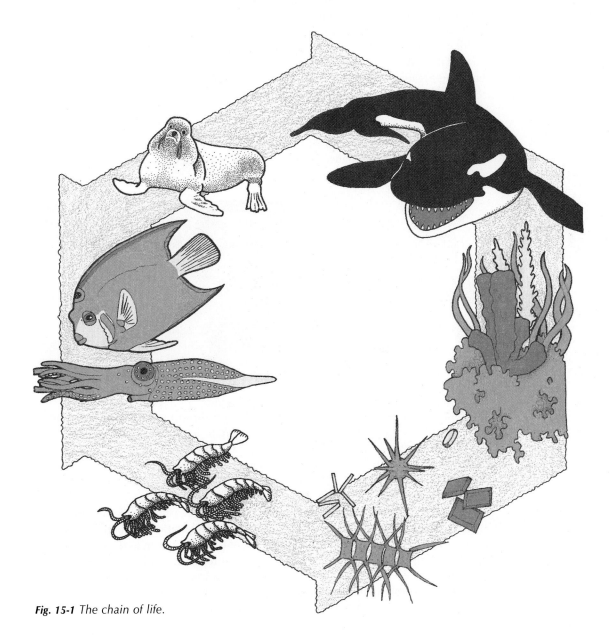

Fig. 15-1 *The chain of life.*

Occasionally, the balance of nature is disrupted by nature itself. Where ideal growing conditions exist, the population of one or more species may increase to huge proportions, far beyond what is considered normal. When this happens, nature tends to rebalance itself. As the population increases, it demands more food. As the food source diminishes from demand, so does the population, until the population and food are once again in balance.

Left undisturbed, nature establishes a system in which the strongest and most fit for the environment survive. The weak are killed and eaten and the survivors produce successive generations which become more adept at survival. This system constantly improves the species.

All through the oceans you can see large and small creatures helping one another. The small crabs discussed in Chapter 13 assist in keeping coral healthy by removing organic debris and consuming it.

The relationship between the sharks and the sharksucker remora is a good example of one fish, which otherwise might serve as food for the other, living peacefully with its potential predator. The remora cleans parasites and other small organisms from the shark's skin. In so doing, it is provided with a food source for itself and assists in the maintenance of the shark's well-being (Fig. 15-2).

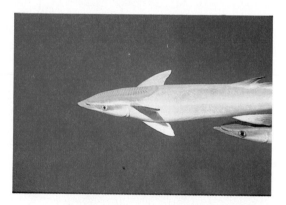

Fig. 15-2 *The remora and shark live in a symbiotic relationship.*

The small cleaner wrasse, other fish, and some shrimp operate cleaning stations throughout the oceans where the larger fish come to have parasites cleaned off their bodies. The larger fish even allow the small creatures to enter their mouths and remove food from their teeth. The cleaners are rewarded with a steady supply of food that they remove from their "clients." These associations, wherein both groups benefit from the relationship, is known as symbiosis.

Man, the ultimate predator, in an effort to provide a better life for himself, is constantly upsetting the balance of nature. The exploitation of natural resources (animal, vegetable, and mineral), the process of construction in and around the water, and the dumping of waste all disturb the natural chain of life in some way.

Nature has an amazing capacity for recovering from disturbances and adapting to change. However, the magnitude and severity of the environmental stresses of modern times are threatening to exceed nature's ability to adapt. Changes in environmental quality affect all creatures in the chain of life and they ultimately affect the quality of life on the *entire* planet.

COASTAL PROBLEMS

Sewage and Garbage

The dumping of improperly treated or untreated sewage and garbage into rivers or immediately offshore into the oceans kills much of the local marine life. The survivors soon show a variety of diseases, and ultimately produce a high degree of mutations (Fig. 15-3). The affected creatures, while not fit for human consumption, are not safe as food for other members of the food chain. Healthy fish that eat the sick are also affected.

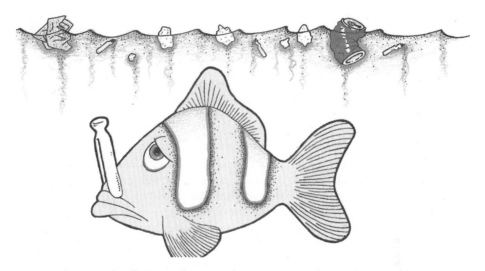

Fig. 15-3 *Sources of pollution endanger and mutate various forms of marine life.*

Pollution, in all its forms, is affecting not only the fish living in the water, but also the people who live around the water and those who make their living from the water (Fig. 15-4). The higher nutrient levels brought about by pollution are thought to be associated with red tide, an algal bloom that causes filter feeders, such as oysters, to become toxic. Solid waste, dumped offshore by municipalities or ships plying waters near the continental United States, may foul the beaches far from its source. Solid waste also affects the recreational potential (swimming, scuba diving, fishing, and boating) of North America's beautiful beaches and coastlines and once-pristine waters.

Many foreign countries have very liberal laws pertaining to the treatment of sewage. The result is the dumping of raw sewage into rivers which eventually flow

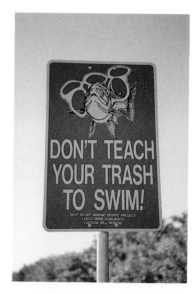

Fig. 15-4 A friendly reminder not to create additional pollution while on or near the water.

to the sea at or near swimming beaches. Swimmers coming in contact with pollution of this kind run a high risk of contracting many diseases, including dysentery and hepatitis.

Construction

Dredging, landfill, and general construction along the shoreline may enhance real estate values but generally degrade the habitats of the shallow-water animals and tend to disturb or destroy the natural food cycle (Fig. 15-5).

Especially vulnerable are the fragile coral reefs and estuaries, both acting as the

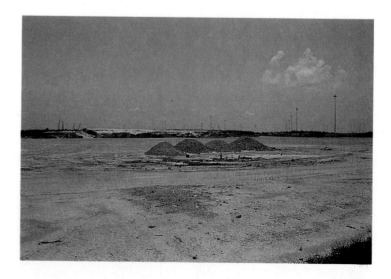

Fig. 15-5 Construction near the water can tend to disrupt the ecosystem and interrupt the cycle of life.

oceans' nurseries. The silt created by dredge-and-fill construction ultimately settles along the reefs and shallow estuaries, killing the coral and young of many species. The deaths of the coral and the associated shallow-water creatures may irreparably upset the chain of life. The ramifications may negatively affect not only animals in the immediate vicinity, but the entire ocean community.

INDUSTRY

Chemical Dumping

Chemical dumping by industry produces much the same results as sewage. It kills the marine life and causes deformation and disease. In fresh water, industrial waste may contaminate the groundwater and decrease the quality of our drinking water. In the southeast, huge underground natural conduits (the aquifer) carry hundreds of millions of gallons of fresh water every day. Contamination of these aquifers in the form of injection wells and uncontrolled storm-water runoff can significantly lower the quality of drinking water for a large portion of the area's population. Ways are currently being developed to monitor the legal disposal of industrial waste and the incidental runoff from agriculture which includes pesticides and herbicides. Fortunately, the U.S. Environmental Protection Agency has strict laws and is enforcing them with heavy fines for offenders. A constant watch must be maintained to avoid illegal or uncontrolled dumping and to monitor the quality of one of our most valuable resources—fresh water.

Crude Oil Damage

Crude oil has caused a great deal of damage to some coastal areas' beauty, recreation, and marine life. Land animals which depend on the sea for their life have suffered, too.

There have been natural crude-oil seepages for millions of years and the oceans

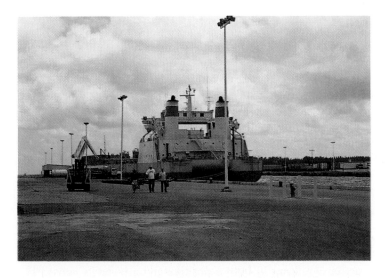

Fig. 15-6 Accidents involving large oil tankers can dump quantities of oil into the ocean which exceed an area's ability to handle the spill.

have handled them effectively. However, with the depletion of our natural oil reserves on land, man has reached into the oceans to tap its riches and resources. Considering the drilling under the sea and the quantity of oil transported on the sea, the potential for spilling more oil than the ocean can handle is significant.

Two major sources of oil spills exist because of the world's thirst for oil. One is the unintentional release of oil from supertankers plying the waters around the world, following a grounding or a collision at sea (Fig. 15-6).

The other source of oil spill is intentional. When oil tankers are transporting their 2 billion tons of oil each year, they carry crude oil one way, then use seawater for ballast on the return voyage. At the end of the return voyage, they dump the seawater along with its oily residue back into the oceans. The oil industry estimates that 5 million tons of oil are disposed of in this manner each year, and scientists estimate that ballast pumping accounts for as much oil pollution as the huge accidental spills which we hear so much about. This dumping is quite legal yet equally tragic from an environmental standpoint.

Commercial Fishing

Pollution, accidental or intentional, is not the only major contributor to the decline of some fish populations. Overharvesting is an equally great threat to their existence. In recent years, sophisticated electronic equipment and satellite photographs have improved the techniques and catches of long-line fishing boats, trawlers, and purse seiners. New, larger boats are able to process the fish as they are caught and can catch and store far beyond what the fishermen of just a few years ago ever dreamed possible.

Even with today's improved fishing techniques, fishing boats in some areas in 1972 were able to take only about 10 percent of the amount harvested in 1965. This trend continues today, and without restraint, many parts of the oceans are being depleted of their available resources.

With the commercial fishing techniques employed today have come the accidental demise of some nonfood species. Dolphins, sea turtles, and other such creatures are occasionally sacrificed in our quest to exploit the oceans more efficiently. Techniques and sophisticated devices are currently being developed to help reduce the numbers of such creatures lost while maintaining a desired level of productivity.

Some forms of sea farming are practical, but not every species can be controlled. Consequently, fishermen must be careful not to deplete the stock of fish beyond chances for natural recovery.

The seas currently provide only a small percentage of animal protein used by the world. If the demand increases, conservation methods will have to be strictly enforced for fishermen throughout the world. It must be remembered that only about one-tenth of the ocean is really fertile—the rest is virtually barren.

SPORT DIVING

The threat to the oceans as a whole by sport divers is minimal. Since the activity of sport divers is limited to the most productive areas of the world's oceans, however, the potential for impact is significant in both a positive and a negative sense. The sport diver has a responsibility to respect and appreciate all aquatic life and not take just for the sake of taking. Spearfishing is fine for food, but to take fish just for sport is unnecessary. The same is true for the taking of crustaceans and shellfish.

For those interested in spearfishing, it is recommended that the proper equipment be practiced with to avoid maiming fish instead of killing them cleanly.

Along the coastal waters of the United States, fish and game departments have established strict limits and seasons which are designed to allow the biomass to maintain itself naturally yet also allow for fishing as a sport.

Sport divers must respect the underwater environment and avoid damaging it. Damage is done in a variety of ways. Intentional damage, probably the most obvious, is done constantly by collectors who pillage the beauty of the reef to sell dead and dried marine life to the public. Accidental damage is just as significant and results from divers who are unable to control their buoyancy, leaving a trail of broken and damaged coral as they traverse a reef.

Divers should strive to minimize their impact on the underwater environment (Fig. 15-7). Do not break off coral or disturb underwater life. Do not remove anything natural unless there is a very good reason. Remember that it took millions of years for the reef to develop and it takes only a few moments to destroy it.

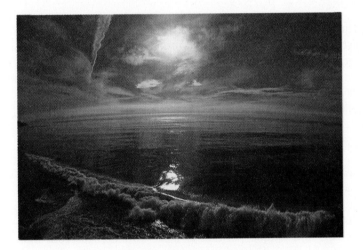

Fig. 15-7 *Divers should approach a clean dive site with the idea that they will "take only memories and leave only bubbles."*

Through the eyes of the diver the world can be made to see the unsurpassed beauty and fragile nature of the underwater world and the wonderful creatures whose home it is. The world below the waves belongs to the marine life there and we humans are just visitors who should leave no evidence of our brief time there. As the environmentally conscientious say, "Take only memories, leave only bubbles."

INLAND PROBLEMS

Problems in fresh water are much the same as in the oceans and include sewage, garbage, and industrial dumping plus additional water-quality problems created by widespread use of insecticides.

Chemical fertilizers and runoff from cattle-feeding and crop-growing operations eventually settle in ponds and lakes. The runoffs are creating a problem known as eutrophication. Eutrophication is a process whereby too many nutrients enter a body of water, causing a sometimes explosive increase in plant growth. As the plants die, they deplete dissolved oxygen in the water and produce lethal methane gas, killing the animal life.

If the intentional or accidental dumping of nutrients is not curtailed, it is only a matter of time until eutrophication begins to take its toll on larger bodies of water, with long-range depletion of fresh-water life as we know it today.

Another problem afflicting fresh waters in the northern half of the United States and Canada is acid rain. As "smokestack" industries have spewed forth substances which form acids when mixed with water vapor in the atmosphere, the results have been rain and snow with increased levels of acids and the bottom-line effect of acid-ifying streams and lakes. The impact of acid rain is recognized by the depletion of once common life forms in lakes and streams. Most notable among the life forms disappearing are what many biologists consider to be environmental barometers— the frogs and salamanders.

SOLUTIONS

It would be a wonderful thing if it were possible to list the causes of pollution, and then, just as easily, list and initiate solutions to the problems. Unfortunately, such is not the case.

The solutions to the pollution problems are at least as complex as the problems themselves. Ecologists are painfully aware that dramatic action to eliminate the obvious may, in fact, create new problems that are equally bad, if not worse.

SUMMARY

One point shines clearly amid the confused quest for answers. Pollution is every-one's problem, and each individual must do his or her part to keep the pollution levels down to a minimum to allow nature to handle it. Until such time as answers are found, a program of public understanding and active prevention must be main-tained. You, the diver, are in a unique position to make a difference. Your first-hand knowledge and experiences can be vital to others less fortunate in understanding the nature of the problem. Do your part to preserve and improve the environment that means so much to us all.

16

Food from Sea and Lake

- Spearfishing
- Abalone
- Conch
- Oysters, Scallops, and Clams
- Fresh-water Shellfish
- Lobsters
- Crabs
- Shrimp
- Commercial Development of the Seas for Food

At the conclusion of Chapter 16, you will be able to:

1. Explain the limitations recommended regarding the taking of fish with a speargun.

2. Describe how fish may react in a reef where spearfishing is common and how that compares to fish in a reef where spearfishing is banned.

3. Name the type of speargun in which the spear and handle are not connected by a line.

4. List four power sources for spearguns.

5. Explain the limitations on spearfishing in certain parts of the world.

6. State where a speargun should be loaded and unloaded.

7. State the considerations when returning undersize abalone.

8. Name the tool used for harvesting abalone.

9. State the limitation on the taking of shellfish, other than legal season.

10. Name the two reasons why a lobster might not be "legal."

Abalone	"Short"	Conch
Dungeness crab	Sea farming	

The seas and lakes provide an important part of our daily food. Often a bountiful array of fish and shellfish inhabit where divers roam.

A careful balance of conservation and harvest is essential to insure productive waters.

Environmentalists have recently made it clear that the seas are showing the adverse effects of regional overfishing. Additionally, commercial interests seem to have a tendency to fish to exhaustion a plentiful supply of a profitable species, and it is not until the supply in a given area is nearly exhausted that steps are taken to manage the harvest.

There is little question that the solutions will involve participation and sacrifices from both commercial and recreational fishermen alike.

The knowledgeable sport diver, using selective techniques and careful conservation, threatens the ecosystem little and may even help it. By abiding by established game laws and conservation practices, and helping others to do the same, a responsible sport diver can change the current adverse conditions into those which allow for a productive future for both the sea and the sport diver.

SPEARFISHING

Though spearfishing has been a popular activity for skin and scuba divers for years, it would be prudent to limit spearfishing activities to killing only those fish that are absolutely necessary for one's own food needs. Killing fish for sport not only may deplete breeding stock but may unbalance the ecosystem as well.

Divers who frequent reefs where spearfishing is prohibited have learned that it is easier to approach fish in those areas, which are not as likely to bolt from any sounds that resemble the discharge of a speargun.

In a reef where spearfishing is common, fish will dart away when any sharp sounds occur. Perhaps fish are not intelligent, but they are conditioned to those things that threaten them, and where spearfishing takes place, sharp sounds condition the response to flee danger.

Spearfishing offers many challenges because the sport diver must function within an environment that belongs solely to the fish.

While spearfishing has little effect in relation to sophisticated commercial trawlers, each diver must do his share to avoid depleting the precious resources from the oceans. Therefore, it is suggested that spearfishing be used only to take food and not for sport, and that careful conservation methods be employed to protect the fish and allow them to reproduce in their own manner.

Techniques and Equipment

The speargun is the most important piece of equipment, and a large variety are available for spearfishing.

The Hawaiian sling resembles a slingshot, with the shaft going through the handle and into a notch attached to the rubber sling. The shaft is free (not connected by line to the handle) and should be used only and may be legal only in salt water where the water is sufficiently clear to keep track of any game that might be speared.

While the Hawaiian sling is efficient, its use is difficult to master. In many parts of the world, the Hawaiian sling is the only spearfishing device allowable and then only while skin diving. It is not permitted when scuba diving.

In addition to the Hawaiian sling, there are a wide variety of guns available including rubber sling guns with single or multiple slings, CO_2-powered guns, spring-powered guns, and pneumatic guns. Selection of speargun type is dependent on the type of game being sought and the surroundings in which one plans to pursue game.

No matter what type of speargun one chooses, it must be treated with respect. Always load and unload the gun in the water away from others and never point it at anyone—it is a potentially dangerous weapon.

The diver, in selecting the type of gun to utilize, should consider the kind of fish to be taken, the area to be hunted, and the potential for ecosystem damage by the weapon chosen.

Choose the type of speargun that will efficiently kill the fish you seek and has an effective range for the type of environment in which the spearfishing will take place. If large fish are being sought, make sure you have sufficient line in the event the fish runs after being shot.

If considering spearfishing in fresh water, it is important to recognize that most parts of the United States and Canada do not permit spearfishing in fresh water. In the few places where fresh-water spearfishing is permitted, many do not allow the taking of game fish with a spear.

SALT-WATER SHELLFISH

Abalone

Many edible shellfish inhabit salt waters. Among the most popular are the abalone. They are excellent food and are found from Alaska to Mexico. Because of their excellent taste, they are in great demand and, as a result, supplies have been depleted drastically. Strict controls have been placed on abalone in U.S. waters.

California, for example, has strict controls over the species and depths at which abalone may be taken and the amount and size which may be captured. In southern California, the sport daily take is limited to two abalone, while commercial fishing is still not limited. Methods of taking abalone are also limited in California, for if undersize (or "short") abalone are taken and discarded or improperly replaced, they will either die or be eaten by predators. They may not be able to replace themselves in their natural habitat of rocks and ledges and could be helpless on the open ocean floor.

You should use a legal abalone iron which is less than 36 inches long; it must be straight or curved with a radius of not less than 18 inches. The iron should be ¾ inch or more wide and ¹⁄₁₆ inch or more thick. It should have no sharp edges. To remove the abalone, slide the iron under it at a 15- to 20-degree angle, while keeping the tip against the rock. Once the iron is under the abalone, lift up on the iron.

If you do remove an undersize abalone, replace it immediately with its foot down against the exact same spot you removed it from.

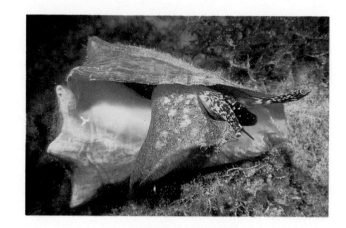

Fig. 16-1 *The conch is another of the more sought after salt-water shellfish.*

Conch

The conch, pictured in Fig. 16-1, is another excellent source of food. It is found crawling along the bottom, primarily in warmer waters. It varies in size from very small to several pounds. While there are a number of species of conch, you cannot eat all of them. It is a good idea to check with the local people to determine which are safe to eat. Also, make certain that you are familiar with all local fish and game regulations and *abide by them!*

Oysters, Scallops, and Clams

The common oyster, scallop, and clam are three more ocean delicacies. Oysters and scallops dwell on rocks, gravel, or mud, while clams are normally found on the bottom, particularly along the shore areas in the mud, or in sand along the beaches. In most parts of the United States you will find that shellfish have minimum legal size limits, so you should familiarize yourself with local regulations. Locating oysters, scallops, or clams varies according to the area. Again, checking with local divers is the best idea.

FRESH-WATER SHELLFISH

The only shellfish found in fresh water in sufficient quantities or large enough to be of interest to divers are fresh-water clams. They live in many lakes throughout the United States and vary in size from 2 to 8 inches in length. Although they are a little tough, they are very tasty. Clams are found on the bottom areas in the bays of lakes and still-water ponds. To determine if the clam is edible, see if it can be opened easily. Clams which cannot be opened easily are usually healthy, and those which can be opened with your fingers may be sick and should be avoided.

SALT-WATER CRUSTACEANS

There are a large number of edible crustaceans found in the oceans. Among these are lobster, crab, and shrimp.

Lobsters

There are two common types of lobster. The spiny lobster lives along the west coast of the United States, down through Mexico, into the Caribbean, and up as far north as Virginia. The spiny lobster lacks the large front claws of the so-called Maine lobster (Fig. 16-2). In hunting lobsters, it is most important to be certain that they meet the legal size limit as specified by local laws and also that the lobster you catch is not an egg-bearing female (Fig. 16-3).

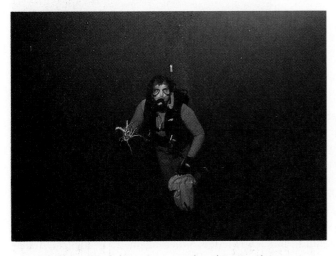

Fig. 16-2 *The spiny lobster is a popular objective for many divers.*

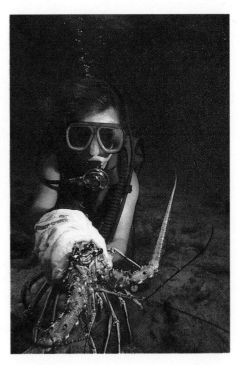

Fig. 16-3 *This diver has successfully captured a legal-size male lobster.*

Crabs

Another delicious crustacean is the crab. Crabs may be found virtually all over the world in one form or another. Not all crabs are edible, and it is strongly suggested that you check rules and regulations with local people regarding the types available. Some crabs and lobsters prefer similar haunts. Fig. 16-4 is a very close look at a huge Caribbean crab in the Gulf of Mexico. However, Dungeness crabs walk upon the sand and silt bottom or bury into the substrate. A careful eye must be kept to locate these deceptive creatures and one must move swiftly to outswim their fast-walking maneuvers.

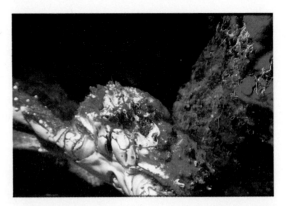

Fig. 16-4 Crabs are difficult to find, but this may be what will confront you when you peer under a coral overhang.

Shrimp

Shrimp are almost totally nocturnal and are rarely seen during the day, but are fascinating sights on a night dive. They range in size from almost microscopic to the size of a small lobster. Shrimp can be found all over the world. They are highly sought after for food. Their numbers, too, appear to be waning.

There are many edible sea creatures besides those already mentioned. Many are considered delicacies, such as sea urchin, turtle, squid, octopus, and a number of others which are not readily available in the commercial market. Each type of animal requires special handling and knowledge. Once again, it is suggested that information from local people regarding rules and regulations be obtained prior to taking any creature unfamiliar to you, and that you carefully observe all applicable regulations regarding taking of underwater game.

COMMERCIAL DEVELOPMENT OF THE SEAS FOR FOOD

There are numerous sea farms cultivating the seas for commercial use. Among the most successful sea farming ventures are turtle and salmon farming and the cultivation of shrimp and oyster beds. Seaweed is being used as a human food supplement as a source of minerals and vitamins. New uses are sought regularly. Attempts to commercially cultivate lobsters have failed so far. This concept appears to be one that fascinates, and this industry will undoubtedly expand in the future.

Dive Planning

17

- Conditioning
- Considerations for Women in Diving
- Dive Objective
- Dive Site Selection
- Scouting the Site
- Equipment Preparation
- Environmental Considerations
- Weather Forecasting
- The Dive Day
- Predicting the Dive Conditions
- The Dive
- After the Dive
- Safe Diving Practices

OBJECTIVES

At the conclusion of Chapter 17, you will be able to:

1. Name the step that is a systematic process of preparing for an open-water diving experience.

2. Describe a quick way to evaluate your state of hydration on the day of a dive.

3. State the recommendation regarding pregnancy and diving.

4. Define the dive objective.

5. Explain how you might scout a dive site if it is a long distance from your home.

6. State an important safety element in scouting a dive site.

7. Name two safety-related pieces of equipment that you might take with you other than dive equipment.

8. Explain why you should begin to check dive equipment earlier than the morning of the dive.

9. Describe when and why you begin to check prevailing weather at a dive site.

10. Complete the statement "Plan your dive and _____ _____ _____."

KEY TERMS

Save-a-dive kit	Complex carbohydrates	Hydration
Plankton bloom	Good visibility	Preparedness

Dive planning is a systematic process of preparing for an open-water diving experience. You and your buddy must consider all aspects of the dive in order to increase safety and enjoyment.

Every dive you make requires some degree of planning and preparation. A dive in a foreign country obviously requires more planning than a local dive to your favorite site; however, *both* require planning. Thorough preparation leads to a relaxed, enjoyable, and successful dive. As the saying goes in competitive athletics, "failure to prepare … is preparing to fail."

In the context of sport diving, a failure in proper dive planning could certainly reduce the enjoyment of the dive but could also seriously compromise the safety of both diver and buddy. Proper planning also takes care of little things that could easily cause the cancellation of the dive. The old adage, "An ounce of prevention is worth a pound of cure" certainly holds true for sport diving. The first time you are at that favorite dive site and break a mask or fin strap, without a replacement, can graphically illustrate the need for preparation and a save-a-dive kit.

However, there is more to dive planning than making sure your equipment is in working order and can handle the rigors of the dive. In addition to having the appropriate level of confidence (in yourself, your buddy, and your equipment) for the dive, you will need to establish a dive objective, select a site, critically evaluate its environment, and develop a plan that will enable you and your buddy to dive within the limits of your training and qualifications. It may seem bothersome, but with a little practice, the positive effects of good dive planning and preparation will ensure that each dive is an enjoyable and safe experience.

CONDITIONING

Physical conditioning should be a regular part of your daily activities, whether you are an active diver or not. If you are in shape, only a slight modification of your exercise routine is needed to prepare you for a dive. Swimming, snorkeling, refresher/requalification pool sessions, and any activity that strengthens and exercises the muscles used while diving are excellent methods of preparing for the dive.

An honest and accurate appraisal of your current physical condition and capability for the physical performance required to cope with the potential physical demands of the dive are vitally important for your safety and well-being (Fig. 17-1). Aerobic capacity, age, weight, drugs, alcohol, and smoking all have a substantial effect on your body's ability to function properly underwater. If you are over age 40, overweight, or have any physical factors which may compromise your safety or your buddy's, a physical examination should be part of your dive preparation. Most entry level scuba programs request a medical statement before training.

Nutrition is also an important factor in preparing for a dive. Foods that are high in fats and oils reduce the ability of the blood to transfer oxygen to your muscles and brain, which can cause muscle cramps, underwater blackouts, and heart attacks. On the other hand, eating complex carbohydrates, such as whole grains, rice, fruit, and vegetables, promotes controlled energy absorption. The night before and the day of your dive, avoid overeating and consuming gas-producing foods.

Hydration prior to a dive is another important health and safety consideration.

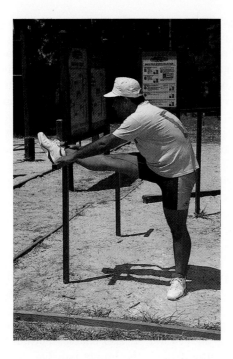

Fig. 17-1 *Good physical conditioning should be a "must" for sport diving.*

Consumption of adequate amounts of water starting early in the evening the night before your dive will help avoid dehydration, thereby reducing the risk of decompression sickness. You will know that you are adequately hydrated if your urine is clear, not colored, before a dive. Between dives, drink sufficient fluids but stay away from those that increase urine output (coffee, cola, tea, and alcohol, for example). Instead, use those which will continue to adequately hydrate you without stimulating increased urine output. Cold water is probably best.

Considerations for Women Divers

Some considerations about health exclusive to women divers deal with pregnancy. It is generally recommended that a pregnant woman, or even one who thinks she might be pregnant, not scuba dive because of the possible (though not proven) harm that the high-pressure environment underwater may have on the fetus. Since the fetus does not have the same filtering mechanism through the lungs that we do, "silent" bubbles that are harmless to the scuba diver might be very dangerous to the fetus.

For women who are not pregnant but are using birth control pills, it is felt that the pill may tend to cause physical changes which make a body slightly more susceptible to decompression sickness. Whether true or not, a conservative use of diving tables can put that concern out of mind.

Other health-related questions posed by women new to diving are about menstrual periods. Experienced women divers respond heartily that diving during their period is physiologically safe and requires only normal sanitary protection. If you are subject to extremely heavy bleeding during your period and experience side effects from the blood loss, be particularly attentive to proper hydration before diving. Otherwise, the menstrual period should be no constraint to diving.

Physiologically, your female reproductive system is not built to trap air, even while using tampons, so it cannot cause an overexpansion problem similar to that which can befall your lungs. Physically, you need no other than your normal precautions for separating your period from the environment, especially since evidence shows that shark and other marine life is *not* attracted by menstrual blood.

There being no known side effects of menstruating while submerged, you are as free to dive as you are to swim, play tennis, or otherwise exert yourself during your period. Always consult your personal physician for advice before taking on scuba training.

DIVE OBJECTIVE

The objective is simply the purpose or reason for the dive. It can be anything from just looking around and enjoying the underwater scenery to photography, spearfishing, or lobstering.

A specific objective ensures that you and your buddy have agreed and are coordinated to do the same thing underwater. It also enables both of you to plan and equip yourselves properly for the dive. If the buddy pair has differing objectives, the dive will surely include confusion and frustration—that is not what safe diving is about.

DIVE SITE SELECTION

Once you have the dive objective firmly in mind, you can get down to the business of researching, selecting, and scouting a dive site, as shown in Fig. 17-2, to match your objectives and qualifications.

To research a potential site, consult your local dive store or a sport diving club, or ask experienced local divers for information and recommendations. Also, obtain information on and select an alternate dive site in case changing conditions make your original site unsuitable. The alternate should be within a reasonable travel time from your primary site and perhaps be in a sheltered area to preclude rough seas or adverse weather conditions from interfering with your dive.

SCOUTING THE SITE

With the site selected, you can begin the process of scouting the dive site. This is basically a search for such information as depths, expected visibility, hazards, local surfs, tides, currents, bottom type and composition, and underwater life. Scouting helps uncover all the pertinent facts about the dive environment you may encounter.

One of the easiest ways to scout the site is to visit it before the dive for a first-hand observation. If this is not possible, you can select one of the various scuba

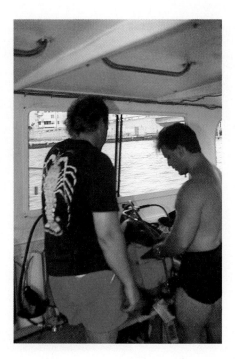

Fig. 17-2 *Evaluating a dive site to compare the site with objectives and diving abilities.*

guidebooks usually found in dive stores, book stores, or libraries. Books often provide the only general descriptions of a dive site, whereas talking to local divers who have actually dived at the spot usually gives detailed data to enhance your dive.

An important element in scouting the site is researching the emergency services available and preparing an emergency plan. This includes emergency contact information such as phone numbers and radio frequencies for the U.S. or Canadian Coast Guard, the local number for local emergency medical services, the nearest medical facility, the nearest functioning recompression chamber, and the best mode of emergency transportation. Another important phone number to have is the Divers Alert Network. DAN is a communication network uniting hyperbaric chambers with divers and their physicians to arrange consultation, transportation, and treatment through a single emergency phone number. DAN provides 24-hour diving medical assistance if you call 919-684-8111 and nonemergency medical and safety advice if you call 919-684-2948 (9 AM to 5 PM EST).

Besides knowing DAN's number, carrying a first-aid kit appropriate for the dive site and knowing how to properly use its contents adds to your emergency plan (Fig. 17-3). Just be sure the kit is checked periodically and restocked after every use.

An additional safety item which you should consider is an oxygen system (Fig. 17-4). If you do not take one to the dive site yourself, at least know where the nearest police, fire, or emergency services station is located to get quick access to oxygen.

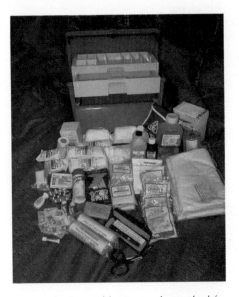

Fig. 17-3 *A first aid kit, properly stocked for diving problems, is only one part of your dive plan.*

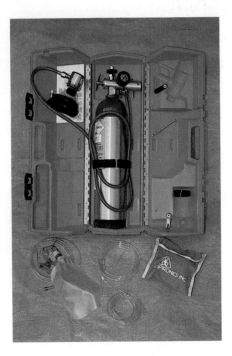

Fig. 17-4 *Safety-conscious divers also include an appropriate oxygen system in their dive-safety equipment and take advantage of courses teaching the proper use of such equipment.*

EQUIPMENT PREPARATION

Now that the dive site is researched, selected, and scouted, you can assemble the appropriate equipment for the dive (Fig. 17-5). Check it all well in advance of the dive day to ensure it works. Taking the time to thoroughly inspect your gear could save you a considerable amount of frustration at the dive site and will definitely reduce inconvenience and possible risk to you and your buddy. It is certainly better to detect a faulty buoyancy compensator while in your living room than at 60 feet on a dive. Begin inspecting early enough so that, if you find any malfunctioning or suspect equipment, you will have ample time to have it serviced or replaced. You and your buddy may take advantage of this opportunity to familiarize yourselves with each other's equipment especially if you have not been diving together recently.

It may be helpful to use an equipment checklist to ensure that nothing is overlooked or forgotten. A comprehensive checklist is included in the Appendix. You can modify the checklist according to your dive objective and site. If you are planning a game-taking trip, your equipment requirements will be different than for a photographic dive.

Take your time at this stage of the planning; your safety, the safety of your buddy, and your enjoyment of the dive will depend upon the proper function and

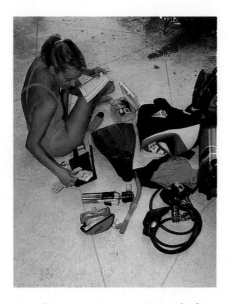

Fig. 17-5 Assembling the equipment well in advance of dive day.

use of your equipment. It might be a good idea for you and your buddy to try out any new or unfamiliar equipment in a pool under supervision before using it in open water for the first time.

The same applies if you are returning to diving after a long absence from the sport. Refresher, refamiliarization, or requalification courses and programs are available through numerous dive shops, schools, and clubs throughout the United States and Canada.

If you are planning a trip outside your country, you might want to have Customs officials inspect and document the serial numbers on all your equipment to avoid having to pay duty when you return from your trip.

Additional equipment that is often overlooked includes your personal car and the boat that you intend to use. It is disappointing to have to call off the whole dive day due to mechanical problems with a car or boat. Even if you are able to dive, the frustration caused by such problems will detract from your enjoyment and possibly cause additional problems as your attention is turned from the dive itself.

ENVIRONMENTAL CONSIDERATIONS

Environmental concerns generally focus on two major areas: the weather and water conditions at the dive site. The evaluation of the weather should be accomplished early enough to allow you to make alternate plans, if necessary, and to avoid any unwanted surprises. Evaluation of water conditions is saved for the day of the dive, and adverse conditions point to the need to always plan for an alternate dive site.

WEATHER FORECASTING

About a week before the dive, start monitoring the weather for your dive site. Local radio and television news programs provide general weather information, and are good for monitoring weather trends. National weather programs, such as *A.M. Weather*, and cable weather are also good sources. The National Oceanic and Atmospheric Administration (NOAA) and the National Weather Service provide continuous radio broadcasts full of facts.

As the week progresses, keep up with the weather. You should start getting more information specifically on the dive site and look for trends in local frontal activity and conditions, such as fog, wind, and so on.

THE DIVE DAY

The morning of the dive you will need to determine the actual and potential factors that will, or could, affect your dive. Start with yourself and your buddy. Ask, "Can my buddy and I cope with the physical and emotional demands that could potentially be placed on us by the type of dive we have planned?" You need to honestly evaluate your physical and emotional preparedness for each and every dive. Scuba diving, although not a fitness activity in itself, does require a certain degree of physical preparation. Make sure you and your buddy are not suffering from any illness, such as an ear infection or chest cold, that could affect your performance during the dive. It is just as important that you are not under the influence of any drugs or alcohol, or suffering from the residual effects of their use.

PREDICTING THE DIVE CONDITIONS

From your efforts in preparation, you should have a good idea of the environmental conditions at the dive site. You can reconfirm the actual weather by contacting a weather-reporting agency, calling someone close to your intended dive site, and by your own observations at the site itself.

Pay close attention to the possibility of storms or fog. These conditions can move in while you are submerged and create a hazardous situation. It is always best to have someone remain in the boat to alert submerged divers of potentially dangerous changes in topside weather conditions. This person should be capable of operating the boat in case pickup of the divers is necessary. A diver recall signal must also be decided upon prior to initiating the dive. This signal can be as simple as rapping the inside of the hull or submerged ladder or dive platform.

As you reach your intended dive area, take a few minutes to assess the existing conditions before you suit up for the dive (Fig. 17-6). Depending on your observations, you may decide to go to an alternate dive site. The conditions to concentrate on in this decision-making step are current, wave action, water visibility, and wind. Obviously, these are interrelated as they affect diving conditions.

Surface currents, tidal currents, wave action, and surge also should be assessed *prior to* suiting up for a dive. These conditions can cause an exhausting dive and can compromise the safety and reduce the enjoyment of the dive. If you decide conditions are not suitable for diving, you will not have to undress as you did not get dressed in the first place.

Good visibility is most often indicated by crystal blue water. Reduced visibility, often indicated by gray or greenish water, can be caused by plankton or suspended silt as a result of high-energy waves and/or a confused sea.

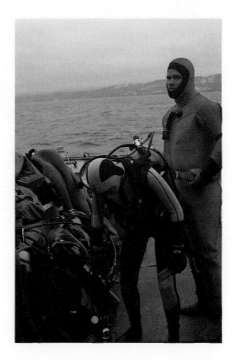

Fig. 17-6 *Looking over the dive site the day of the dive.*

Wind can cause rough surface conditions and upwelling. A strong off-shore wind can cause surface water to flow away from the shore and be replaced by colder water from beneath. When this nutrient-rich bottom water is warmed, an ideal situation exists for the development and growth of plankton. A plankton bloom can severely reduce visibility.

In general, conditions which indicate good diving are light surf with low-energy waves and a time interval between waves to allow a reasonable entry, plus the absence of currents. If there is a current, it should be timed to be favorable to the end of the dive. A calm surface without large waves is the sign of little or no surge. Crystal blue water with bright sunshine provides good visibility and underwater illumination.

If your predive observation reveals good conditions, you are in luck. Before you make the dive, however, ensure that someone not involved in the dive knows your dive plan. This surface support person should know when you expect to return, what to do, and whom to contact if you do not return.

THE DIVE

The final check before entering the water includes a physical inspection and familiarization with each other's equipment, a quick review of the depth and time limits of the dive, observing the sea and current conditions, discussing the kind of descent you will use (free or following an anchor or descent line), setting your watches, and any other points that will have a bearing on the success or enjoyment of the dive (Fig. 17-7).

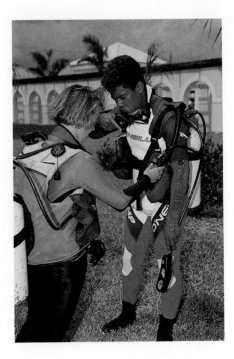

Fig. 17-7 *The predive check that takes place immediately before the dive.*

Many divers conduct safety drills prior to commencing a dive to promote skill familiarity and compatibility between buddies. These "S" or safety drills may include review and practice of procedures to handle safety-related problems, such as out-of-air emergencies, lost diver, rescue, and a quick review of traditional and regional hand signals you intend to use to communicate underwater.

A dive plan is of little value if it is not followed. Preceding the dive, a lot of time and effort went into gathering equipment, information, and people together to insure a pleasant, successful dive. Use your dive plan and follow it closely. The real satisfaction from scuba diving is having a safe, worry-free dive that comes from preparing and following a dive plan. To avoid confusion and promote safety, "Plan your dive and dive your plan!"

AFTER THE DIVE

With the dive completed, it is time to sit back, relax, and relive its exciting moments. If repetitive dives are planned, it is the time to determine your repetitive dive group and update your dive profile. Then, complete your logbooks, inspect your dive equipment and, if necessary, perform any on-site maintenance.

Between dives, keep your preparedness up for subsequent dives; do not ingest any alcohol or drugs, and do not take a hot shower or exhaust yourself with excessive surface interval activities. Such activities will also increase your circulation and promote the formation of nitrogen bubbles. The result could give the symptoms of the bends even though you may have returned to the surface from the previous dive asymptomatic.

A dive that is safe, relaxed, and fun does not just happen; it is planned. The time you spend planning a dive is well worth the effort. It gives you the opportunity to answer questions while you have time to research and resolve them logically. So, when the urge to explore the underwater world strikes, take a moment to gather all the available resources, apply the principles of good dive planning and common sense, use a checklist like the one shown in the Appendix, and follow the safe diving practices below. This moment will help make each dive an enjoyable, successful, and safe experience.

SPORT DIVER STANDARDS FOR SAFE DIVING

As a safe diver, I should:

Dive within my mental and physical limits

Be aware of the need for good physical conditioning in connection with scuba diving

Be aware of the effects of drugs, alcohol, tobacco, and fatty foods on my personal diving safety

Cancel dives when my physical condition or that of my buddy is questionable

Dive within the limits of my training and experience

Always dive with a certified and equally qualified buddy

Have an emergency plan prepared and at the dive site

Avoid excessive hyperventilation when breath-hold diving

Descend slowly and equalize my ears prior to and frequently during descent

Ascend no faster than 60 feet per minute but more appropriately no more than 40 feet per minute

Conduct a safety stop with my buddy at 20 feet to 30 feet for 3 to 5 minutes after every dive

Be familiar with the dive tables and know how to use them

Be conservative with the dive tables

Plan the dive and follow the dive plan

As a safe diver, I should:

Have cylinders hydrostatically tested at least once every 5 years

Have cylinders visually inspected annually

Use only clean, filtered air from an appropriate scuba fill station

Be aware that depth gauges are sometimes inaccurate, and have them tested periodically

Use proper and well-maintained equipment for all planned dives

Have my regulator and other safety devices checked and tested periodically

Know my boat and appropriate boating regulations

Use a diver's flag and surface support

Have a submersible pressure gauge to monitor tank air pressure

Dive with an alternate air source

Wear a buoyancy control device

Use an inflator on my BC

Have a dive timing device

Ensure that the weight belt is not impeded by other equipment

As a safe diver, I should:

Always test all my scuba equipment for proper fit/function

Plan my dive according to seas, actual weather, weather forecast, and my current physical condition

Have a dive plan that includes where and how to obtain emergency assistance

Be familiar with the dive site and determine if it is a beginner or advanced site

Cancel dives when environmental conditions are questionable

Avoid touching anything underwater that may be alive

Remove any game killed in the water as soon as possible

Obey all local fish/game rules

Restrictions: As a safe diver, I should:

Dive often

Never let an uncertified diver use my equipment

Never scuba dive with individuals who are not certified

Be aware of the effects of nitrogen narcosis on my ability to make judgments

Obtain an orientation before diving in an unfamiliar area

Avoid dives below 100 feet

Dive review: As a safe diver, I should:

Strive to improve my diving knowledge by attending diving educational seminars and conventions

Make one or more reviews with a scuba instructor if it has been over 12 months since my last scuba dive, and have my logbook signed to show that I have dived within 12 months and I am competent in my scuba skills

Good citizen: As a safe diver, I should:

Be familiar with and obey all local diving laws

Be a good sportsman and obey all fish and game laws

18

Specialty Diving

- Cave Diving
- Cavern Diving
- Ice Diving
- Wreck Diving
- Treasure Hunting
- Blue-Water Diving
- Search and Rescue

OBJECTIVES

At the conclusion of Chapter 18, you will be able to:

1. Name the two general requirements of all of the specialties presented in this chapter.
2. Tell what most manmade caves were originally.
3. Name the stone in which most natural caves are found.
4. Explain the ultimate destination of a spring run.
5. Describe the major risk involved in sinkhole diving.
6. Explain how certain caverns may be explored using the "no lights rule."
7. Tell the minimum number of people who must be involved in a safe ice dive.
8. Tell how to avoid potential legal problems after recovering artifacts while wreck diving.
9. Explain the simple definition of blue-water diving.
10. Name the national organization you may contact for additional information and standards regarding search and recovery diving.

KEY TERMS

Sink holes	Lava tubes	Sea caves
Spring side	Siphon side	Guidelines
Cavern	Trapeze	SAR

Part of the fascination toward diving stems from the fact that it provides such a wide range of activity. We have already explored the various hobbies that may be incorporated into the diving picture. Let us now look at some special diving activities that require a good deal more training and expertise than normal diving in open water.

Cave diving, cavern diving, ice diving, blue-water diving, wreck diving, treasure diving, and search and rescue all require their own special brand of excellence. Each represents special diving conditions that introduce additional hazards the open-water diver generally does not have to face. Specialized diving equipment is necessary to provide a reasonable margin of safety for all of these specialized activities.

This chapter offers ideas on how to become involved in something more than just open-water diving. It *is not intended to provide the technical means to participate in these specialized activities*. If you plan to participate in any of them, obtain special training from experts first, for your own safety and enjoyment.

CAVE DIVING

Caves have always been irresistible to people. From the time when people lived in caves, they have always had the desire to explore what is there, way back in the hidden reaches. With the advent of scuba diving, it is now possible to pursue those desires underwater.

Underwater caves can be found all over the world. In the United States, the greatest concentration is in the southeast. Florida is probably the best known area for cave diving and for promoting cave-diving training and safety along with cave diving itself.

Types of Underwater Caves

Caves are classified into several categories: manmade caves, such as abandoned mines and quarries; natural springs and sinkholes; lava tubes; sea caves; and coral caves.

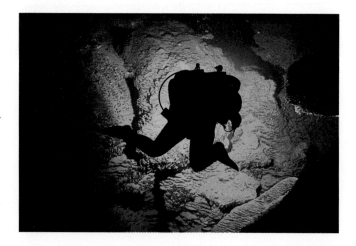

Fig. 18-1 Manmade caves include abandoned mines.

Many manmade caves were originally dry mines that filled with water after they were abandoned, as shown in Fig. 18-1. A sinkhole is created naturally by an underground river flowing near the surface and having its ceiling cave in to create a hole down to the water's surface (Fig. 18-2). Springs are basically underground rivers bubbling to the surface.

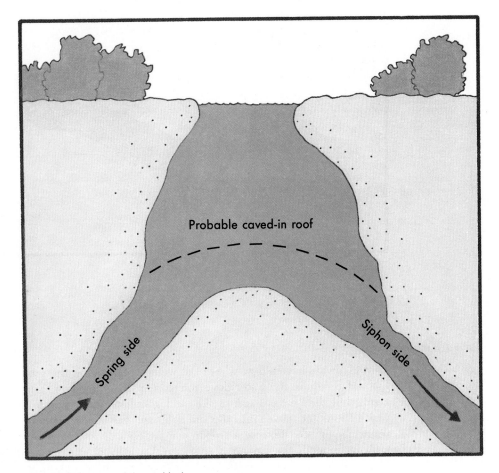

Fig. 18-2 *Diagram of the sinkhole.*

While most natural caves form in limestone, they are found in other types of rock as well (Fig. 18-3). Lava tubes form when volcanoes erupt, and the lava flowing out underwater cools on the outside to form a natural tunnel, with lava flowing within. When the lava flow stops, the tubes flood, making them divable. Sea caves are carved by strong surf beating against the softer layers, or cracks or fractures in the rocky shoreline. The tops of coral reefs may grow together, forming coral caves that may be several hundred feet long.

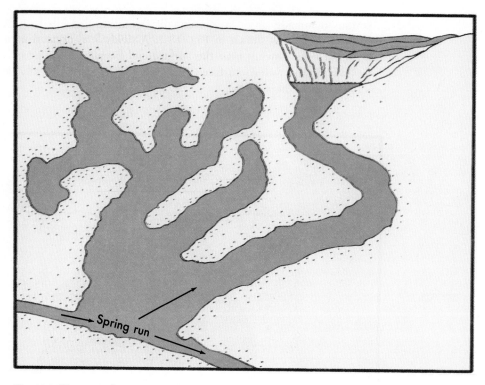

Fig. 18-3 *Diagram of cave.*

Cave Characteristics

Springs always have a flow where the water comes out of the ground, and a run on the surface where the water flows to create a stream or river. Sinkholes never have a run, but they have a spring side and a siphon side. The spring is the point at which the water moves into the sinkhole, and the siphon is the point at which the water moves out. Because a siphon can sweep a diver away from the opening and into the ground, the siphon is considered worthy of attention and is viewed as a high-risk diving environment requiring special training and equipment (Fig. 18-4).

In both caves and springs, there may be many different passages, forming an underwater maze. The diver attempting to exit from the cave without a previously laid guide (safety) line is liable to encounter any number of passages that appear to be exits, but are actually dead ends or routes farther underground.

The floors of most caves are covered with sediment, which is often a very fine silt. When disturbed, it can completely block your vision and hide the exit. Guidelines, properly used, are the *only* way to insure your safe return to the exit. Because they are so essential to the safe completion of a cave dive, guidelines are used even in simple caves to provide you the way out should you be in complete darkness because of silt or loss of lights.

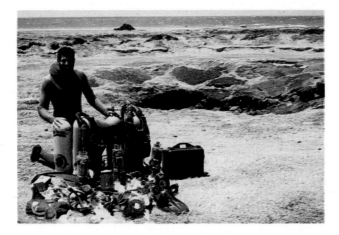

Fig. 18-4 *Cave diving is particularly equipment intensive, as this photo of a cave diver's equipment will attest.*

Attitude and Training

A strong mental attitude is required, because of the real possibility of a safe dive turning hazardous with a flick of a fin or failure of some lights. If that happens to a cave diver who has the wrong mental attitude, it could spell disaster for the diver and the buddies.

Because of the darkness, the lack of access to surface air, and the sheer uncertainty of what lies ahead in caves, much special training and equipment are required. Seek out and obtain professional cave-diving training and all appropriate equipment *before* you enter your first cave.

Training for cave diving is based on the safety rules developed for the activity. These rules are:

1. Be trained for cave diving.
2. Always use a continuous guideline to the surface.
3. Save at least two-thirds of your initial air supply for exiting.
4. Dive no deeper than 130 linear feet.
5. Carry at least three lights per dive.

Cave diving can be a great joy and thrill, despite its requirements. Caves may contain all sorts of attractions, from fossils and antiques to new species of life. The thrill of exploration and the search for the contents of caves is endless. The achievement of conducting a safe, enjoyable cave dive is a tribute to a diver's planning and diving skills.

More information and training in cave diving may be obtained from:

National Speleological Society—Cave
   Diving Section (NSS-CDS)
P.O. Box 950
Branford, FL 32008-9050

National Association for Cave Diving
   (NACD)
P.O. Box 14492
Gainesville, FL 32604

CAVERN DIVING

Cavern diving offers many of the same rewards that cave diving does but without the risk of being out of sight of the entrance. Cavern diving may be safely participated in with minimal additions to your open-water diving equipment, and with much less additional training.

A cavern differs from a cave in that the diver explores the area near the entrance (Fig. 18-5). In order to be considered a cavern, the following environmental constraints must not be exceeded:

1. Natural daylight must be visible from the entrance. Thus there is no cavern diving at night, as there is no sunlight.
2. The divers must remain within 130 linear feet of the surface at all times during the dive.
3. No restrictions may be passed through; a restriction is any place too narrow for the dive team to negotiate easily while swimming side by side.
4. The water visibility must be at least 40 feet.
5. The maximum depth is limited to 70 feet.
6. No decompression diving is permitted.

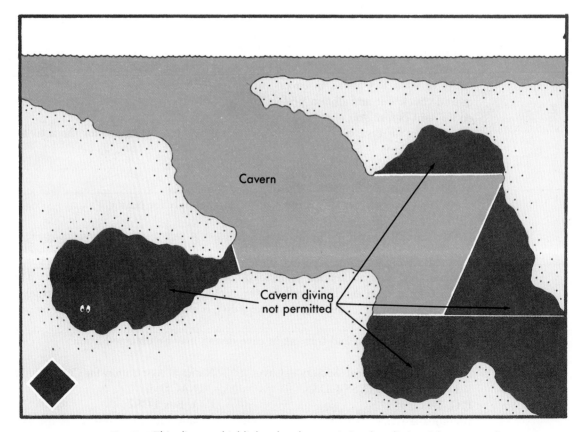

Fig. 18-5 This diagram highlights the characteristics that distinguish a cavern from a cave.

If any of these parameters are exceeded, then the dive is considered a cave dive, requiring full cave-diving gear and training.

While cavern diving does require additional equipment and training, a limited form of cavern diving may be participated in using standard open-water gear. By invoking the "no lights rule" (no diver in the team may carry any dive lights on the dive), a dive team may explore a cavern with reduced risk to themselves. Not having any lights insures that they will not be led away from sight of the entrance by a light illuminating a far-away attraction. This rule may be used only in caverns with only one entrance or opening for light to enter.

ICE DIVING

Diving under the ice is very much like cave diving, except that it is colder. It requires similar equipment (Fig. 18-6). The diver has only one exit and must use safety lines. Because snow often covers the ice, it may be very dark, and lights are normally required.

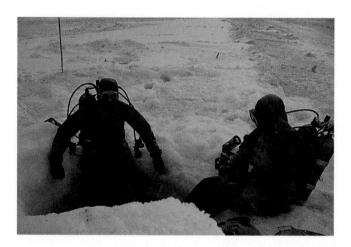

Fig. 18-6 *The equipment and attire for ice diving.*

Ice diving has a special appeal to the adventuresome diver. It can be done wherever ice forms over water deep enough to dive in. There is the natural fascination to wonder what goes on beneath the ice; however, there is little reason beyond the adventure to go ice diving. While the water is sometimes clearer under the ice, there is little to see, because in cold weather most fish hibernate.

Requirements

In bodies of fresh water, water temperatures will range from 32° F to 39° F (0° to 4° C). In ice-covered oceans, temperatures will drop to 28° F (−2° C), since salt water freezes at lower temperatures than fresh water. Air temperatures in the same areas can drop to more than −100° F with wind chill.

In many ways ice diving is even more dangerous than cave diving. The cold does strange things to your mind, to your body, and to your equipment. The cold slows down the bodily functions, so the mind is not able to react quickly to any problem that might arise, and when it does react, there is a physical slowdown that keeps the body from performing needed tasks as well as it does normally. In addition, the equipment is subject to freezing and requires special maintenance and care to keep it in top condition.

The environment below the ice is hostile and requires that a diver prepare for survival. A diver should begin by diving in particularly cold water, learning how to function effectively both mentally and physically. The diver's equipment probably requires special attention to ensure that the air in the tank and regulator is dry enough to prevent condensation and freezing during use. The regulator should be environmentally protected, and the tank is filled with dry air. The air must be totally dry to prevent moisture which might enter from later condensing and then freezing inside the regulator during the dive. While wet suits may be used, dry suits are usually better for comfort and safety. Whichever is used, suits must be in near-perfect condition.

Extra thermal layers may be used to prevent excessive heat loss. When adding extra layers, the diver should have additional practice time in the open water to adapt to the extra equipment. If a dry suit is used, training in its features plus several open-water familiarization dives will prepare the diver for using it under ice.

Safety Precautions

Extra safety precautions are taken prior to ice diving. Safe ice diving is done in two teams of two divers each, plus at least two tenders. The two divers in the water use the buddy system, while two safety divers wait on the surface. Safety lines are attached to the divers in the water and to the safety divers. Since there is little time for trying to determine what was meant by that last tug on the rope, all divers and tenders involved should have a complete knowledge of and be thoroughly drilled in procedures and signals. A wrong interpretation or slow reaction during the dive could spell disaster.

If you are interested in ice diving, it is suggested that you seek an established ice-diving unit. In most areas of the United States where ice diving has been going on for some time, there are people who have established good safety techniques which reduce dangerous possibilities to a minimum. These ice divers can provide the special training and information required to ice dive in safety.

WRECK DIVING

Wreck diving fascinates almost all open-water divers. The mystery and solitude of a wreck must be experienced to be appreciated. Wreck diving may be conducted in salt water or fresh water, on small boats or large ships, and may include recently sunken vessels or old wrecks with great historical value (Fig. 18-7).

Special training is appropriate because wreck diving is very much like cave diving. Water conditions can be quite poor, with the water dirty, and, in the ocean particularly, almost always moving and often quite deep.

When entering a wreck, a prudent diver must be especially aware of internal decay. Even steel ships have a great deal of wood inside them which rots after a

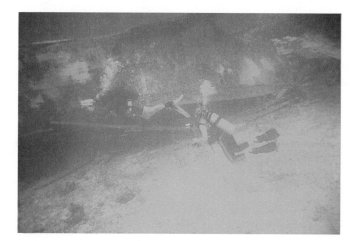

Fig. 18-7 Here divers explore a sunken wreck—a piece of maritime history.

period of time. Sometimes that rotting wood requires nothing more than a diver brushing against it to cause it to collapse.

Wrecks have long been favorite targets for divers. They combine adventure with the search for history, and there is always the lure of treasure. Some divers are interested in only the more commercial possibility of salvage, while others are concerned with purely archeological pursuits.

Whatever your reason for wreck diving, prior to making a dive, learn about the wreck itself. Learn about wreck-diving techniques, and learn about any special techniques particularly required by that wreck. To avoid any possible danger and to ensure the dive will be a success, have your equipment up to par and have the necessary safety equipment.

Prior to removing anything from the water, find out about your legal rights to items you have found. In some areas, there are strict laws in effect which specify the diver's rights; in others it is "finders, keepers." In fresh water, for instance, the prior owner retains ownership at all times, so finding something does not automatically make it yours. Avoid any legal problems that might come up and establish your rights beforehand with the proper authorities.

TREASURE HUNTING

The finding of sudden riches has been one of man's dreams from the beginning of time, and it has also been one of his great joys. Underwater treasure hunting is no different, and great riches have been taken from the seas and rivers.

Treasure does not always come in the form of precious metals, although that is how we normally think of it. It may, in fact, come in the form of artifacts. It may mean prospecting. Many divers are involved in dredging for gold in streams and rivers in parts of the United States where gold is known to exist.

While wreck diving for treasure involves a great deal of expense and research time, prospecting can be done on a very small budget. The rewards are more predictable if not more dramatic.

BLUE-WATER DIVING

Blue-water diving is conducted where the bottom is deeper than safe diving limits. In fact, the water may be several miles deep where this type of diving is conducted. Because of this, good buoyancy control skills are required for safety.

Blue-water diving has allowed researchers to study planktonic life that lives in

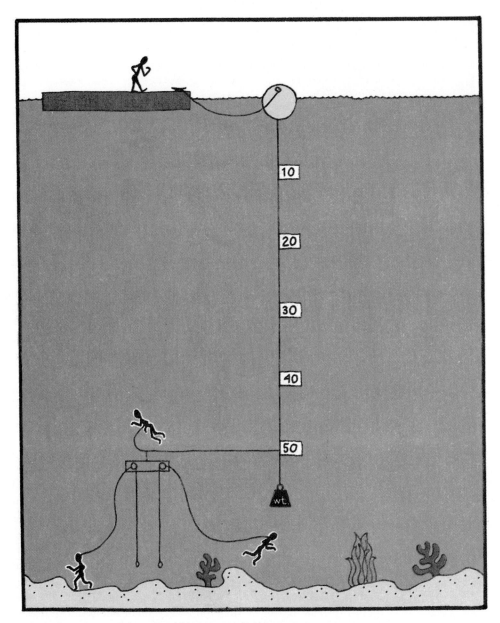

Fig. 18-8 *Drawing of the typical blue-water diving support setup.*

the open ocean. It has also provided divers the means to observe pelagic marine life such as whales, sharks, ocean sunfish, and game fish.

This advanced specialty requires considerable support equipment (Fig. 18-8). Diving takes place from a small boat, which is always manned by a surface support person. A down line from a float provides a visual reference for the divers to prevent disorientation caused by the lack of a visual reference such as the bottom. All divers are attached to the down line using tether lines. The tethers are attached to a trapeze, which allows the lines to play in and out as the divers swim about. A safety diver is positioned at the trapeze to prevent the lines from tangling, and to maintain a visual lookout for hazardous marine life such as sharks.

Blue-water diving should be participated in only after several training dives have been conducted in water with a visible bottom. These dives allow the divers to become familiar with the equipment, practice specialized line communications, practice midwater buoyancy control, and learn their individual dive responsibilities and tasks.

SEARCH AND RESCUE

More and more cities, counties, and states are establishing search and rescue (SAR) units. These groups have been organized to take care of the least pleasant job in diving, but it is a job that must be done, and it must be done safely.

Water accidents invariably occur during the worst conditions. The water is often dirty, deep, cold, or moving. The bottom may contain plant life. The accident could happen at night, but, regardless, rescue always seems to be needed under the worst conditions.

Besides the problem of diving in bad conditions, emotional problems often follow in handling survivors, organizing the searchers, and maintaining order during and after the rescue. The team efforts may not always involve rescue; they may involve recovery when it is too late for rescue.

First aid training is a necessary part of a rescue diver's education as is a general knowledge of emergency techniques.

Search and rescue diving does not appeal to everyone. Those who wish to become involved can contact their local law enforcement authorities, who can put them in touch with the people in charge of local search and rescue or recovery teams in their area.

On the national level in the United States, the National Association for Search and Rescue (NASAR) provides guidelines for organizing and conducting SAR activities. They have a technical committee that specializes in water SAR activities. They may be contacted for further information at:

NASAR
P.O. Box 3709
Fairfax, VA 22038

19 *Careers*

- Sport Diving Instruction
- Journalism
- Photography
- Light Commercial Work
- Heavy Commercial Work
- Sciences

OBJECTIVES

At the conclusion of Chapter 19, you will be able to:

1. Name one aspect of journalism that would be of interest to scuba diving instructors.
2. Name two markets for scuba adventure journalism.
3. State the first step in learning underwater photography.
4. Name two potential buyers for underwater photography.
5. State two attributes of the light commercial diver.
6. Name the biggest plus and the biggest minus of heavy commercial diving.
7. Name the agency which exists and exempts scientific diving from regulation by the Occupational Safety and Health Administration.
8. Name the science applied to the marine environment.
9. Name the science involving the application of sciences to fresh water.
10. Name the science involved in the study of groundwater.

KEY TERMS

Photojournalism

Hard hat rigs

Limnology

Saturation diving

American Academy of Underwater Sciences

Hydrology

Closed-circuit

Oceanography

Archeology

Diving is considered by millions as the most fascinating and exciting of sports, unique in its flexibility and diversity. It requires careful thought, complete training, and keen intelligence to be performed safely. It provides ample sources of recreation, allowing a diver to combine many of the land sports and hobbies that might normally be engaged in with water activities.

For many, diving represents a way to earn a living at something they really love. The employment opportunities in diving fall into four categories: sport diving, which includes instruction and such things as writing and photography; light commercial work, which can be accomplished with scuba gear; heavy commercial work, which requires mixed gas and/or hard-hat gear; and scientific research, which applies any of the sciences to either oceans or fresh waters.

Whatever underwater employment you choose, you are in continual contact with nature, on the threshold of earth's last frontier. You are a real pioneer and part of the world's future.

SPORT DIVING

There are several ways to earn a living in sport diving. Among these are teaching, writing, and photography.

Instruction

The first step in becoming a diving instructor is, of course, sport diver certification. After gaining further diving experience and experience instructing, perhaps as an assistant instructor, you would attend an instructor certification course. These courses are offered by a number of local, national, and international schools and organizations as listed below.

Instructor certification courses last from several days to several weeks. They involve intensive learning experiences in the classroom and in open water and have extremely high standards and rigorous testing procedures.

Some instructor training centers offer student instructors a course not only in diving instruction, but also in retail salesmanship, equipment repair, and all aspects of effective dive store operation. Complete diver education programs (including those for store-oriented and independent instructors) are offered by the National Association of Scuba Diving Schools (NASDS), the National Association of Underwater Instructors (NAUI), the Professional Association of Diving Instructors (PADI), Scuba Schools International (SSI), and the YMCA National Scuba Program.

For specific details, admission, and course information regarding instructor certification schools, write to the following:

International Diving Educators Association (IDEA)
P.O. Box 17374
Jacksonville, FL 32245

Los Angeles County Underwater Instructors Association (LACO)
419 East 192nd Street
Carson, CA 90745

Multinational Diving Educators Association (MDEA)
P.O. Box 3433
Marathon Shores, FL 33052

National Association of Scuba Diving Schools (NASDS)
P.O. Box 17067
Long Beach, CA 90807

National Association of Underwater Instructors (NAUI)
P.O. Box 14650
Montclair, CA 91763

National YMCA Scuba Program
6083-A Oakbrook Parkway
Norcross, GA 30092

Professional Association of Diving Instructors (PADI)
P.O. Box 15550
Santa Ana, CA 92705

Professional Diving Instructors Corporation (PDIC)
1015 River Street
Scranton, PA 18505

Scuba Schools International (SSI)
2619 Canton Court
Fort Collins, CO 80525

NASE, National Academy of Scuba Educators
1728 Kingsley Avenue, Suite 105
Orange Park, Florida 32073 USA
(800) 728-2262

Journalism

As interest in diving grows, so does the demand for information. Journalism and photography offer fields where the diver can convert findings, adventures, and knowledge into money, while enjoying the sport (Fig. 19-1).

Journalistic areas open to the potential writer are education, adventure, and travel.

Education

Instructors everywhere are hungry for technical information. They are constantly in need of information regarding new techniques and in how other instructors are handling problems that arise in training safe divers. In addition, they need information regarding equipment modification and evaluation because few can personally purchase and evaluate each piece of equipment on the market. Written information on these subjects and others of interest to instructors is published not only by the training agencies, but also by popular publications.

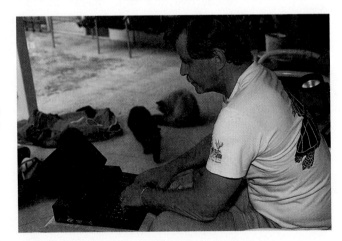

Fig. 19-1 *Journalism is one of the fields open to those interested in and capable in scuba diving.*

Adventure

Every sport has its fictional heroes, and diving is no exception. Stories, both fact and fiction, are in demand for magazines and books since every dive is an adventure. Perhaps your special adventure can be polished into excellent reading.

Travel

Travel information about different diving areas is included in almost every diving publication, even equipment catalogs. Even if a dive resort has already been publicized or reviewed, the appearance of something new could make it worthy of a revisit and retelling. Divers like to read about where to go and what to look for, including any special problems that might shape a vacation and how to handle them.

Photography

Photography is probably the best way other than diving to present the underwater world to other individuals. Photographs are used extensively to highlight articles and stories.

Underwater photographic training begins with a basic photography course on land, perhaps at one of the schools in the United States that specializes in photography. Once the basics of shooting photographs is mastered, they can be translated into underwater techniques by training at most diving equipment stores or with an independent instructor. After gaining experience by exposing several rolls of film underwater, specialized training can be obtained from any of several underwater photography schools. In photography, especially that done underwater, there is no substitute for experience.

For further information see the section on underwater photography in the *Advanced Manual*.

Almost every publication and television station is a potential buyer of underwater pictures. A career in journalism and photography can begin with the basic scuba training you received at your local dive store.

LIGHT COMMERCIAL WORK

Light commercial work is normally defined as underwater work accomplished in a short amount of time or in shallow enough water so that decompression is unnecessary. It generally involves inspection of dams, pipelines, cables, and even sewage outfalls. It may also consist of such things as salvaging small boats, minor underwater repair, boat-bottom cleaning, and even some forms of underwater construction.

To the diver with an imagination, there is an almost endless array of jobs that can be completed with the use of scuba. However, every other certified diver is a potential competitor and, unless there is a big demand in your area, it may not be a dependable source of income.

A competent light commercial diver needs advanced training and a keen mechanical ability. A light commercial worker must be a jack-of-all-trades, skilled at construction techniques, with a good sound knowledge of physics and photography.

Advanced scuba training for light commercial work is available at your local professional school and, of course, on the job. Again, following training, there is no substitute for experience.

HEAVY COMMERCIAL WORK

Heavy commercial work is the highest paid and most hazardous of all commercial diving. Most work is done under adverse conditions where visibility is zero and water temperature is low.

The work involves salvage, repair, maintenance, and construction, and may include saturation diving. Salvage work is normally done on ships or other items worth recovering. Repair, maintenance, and construction work may involve structures such as oil rigs, piers, bridges, dams, and sea walls.

Commercial diving equipment has become quite sophisticated, including closed-circuit scuba and hard-hat rigs that utilize both compressed air and mixed gases.

Before applying to a commercial diving school, you should be thoroughly trained in scuba so you have a good idea of what to expect in heavy commercial work with all its inherent conditions. Commercial instruction usually includes underwater welding, the use of hard hat and mixed gas units as well as heavy construction techniques, plus a lot of hard work.

In the United States, both light and heavy commercial diving is regulated by the Occupational Health and Safety Administration.

SCIENCES

It has already been stated that the waters of the world are our last frontier on earth. Diving is one of the tools used by scientists to examine the happenings in the underwater world personally. More sciences now recognize the potential of the oceans and fresh waters. It is quite apparent that additional research must be done to allow us to tap that great potential.

In order for scientific diving activities in the United States to be exempt from Occupational Health and Safety Administration regulations, the diving operations must comply with the standards of the American Academy of Underwater Sciences, or their equivalent. For further information regarding AAUS, you may write to them:

American Academy of Underwater
   Sciences
947 Newhall Street
Costa Mesa, CA 92627

Oceanography

When science is applied to the marine environment, it is known as oceanography; the scientists are oceanographers. Specializations in oceanography include biology, botany, zoology, geology, geography, and archeology, to name a few. Universities

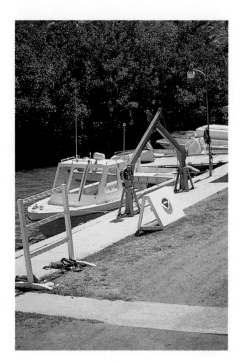

Fig. 19-2 *Scientific research vessels at a National Oceanic and Atmospheric Administration (NOAA) facility in the Caribbean.*

and research institutions of many nations have research vessels operating on the oceans (Fig. 19-2). They employ sophisticated equipment in the form of submersibles, one atmosphere diving systems (OMADS) and remotely operated vehicles (ROVs) in their efforts to unlock the mysteries of the deep.

Limnology

Limnology is the application of the sciences to fresh water as opposed to the marine environment; just as there is a growing need for oceanographers, there is a need for limnologists. The fresh waters, like the oceans, hold a key to our future.

Other areas of interest in underwater research involve hydrology (the study of groundwater resources) and archeology (the study of history). A significant amount of current research concerns pollution and the strains it places upon the oceans of the world. Giant steps are being taken toward locating and stopping the causes of pollution.

If you are interested in a career in the sciences, you must begin with a good background in the science of your choice. It is never too early or too late to start. Junior and senior high school science courses can provide you with the necessary preparation for college study. A college education and degree is an absolute "must" for anyone seeking a career in the sciences. For specific information, contact your local high school or university admissions office for specific information about beginning a career in oceanography or limnology.

Appendix

WATER TEMPERATURE PROTECTION CHART

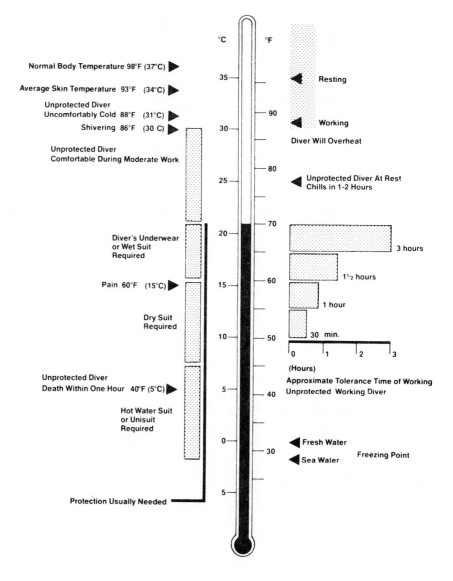

Normal Body Temperature 98°F (37°C) ▶

Average Skin Temperature 93°F (34°C) ▶

Unprotected Diver
Uncomfortably Cold 88°F (31°C) ▶

Shivering 86°F (30 C) ▶

Unprotected Diver
Comfortable During Moderate Work

Diver's Underwear
or Wet Suit
Required

Pain 60°F (15°C) ▶

Dry Suit
Required

Unprotected Diver
Death Within One Hour 40°F (5°C) ▶

Hot Water Suit
or Unisuit
Required

Protection Usually Needed

°C

35

30

25

20

15

10

5

0

5

°F

90

80

70

60

50

40

30

◀ Resting

◀ Working

Diver Will Overheat

◀ Unprotected Diver At Rest
Chills in 1-2 Hours

3 hours

1½ hours

1 hour

30 min.

0   1   2   3

(Hours)

Approximate Tolerance Time of Working
Unprotected Working Diver

◀ Fresh Water

◀ Sea Water   Freezing Point

AIR PURITY STANDARDS

The U.S. Navy Diving Manual provides that air used in scuba operations must meet minimum standards of purity as established by the Commander Naval Medical Command. The standards applied by the U.S. Navy are as follows:

Oxygen concentration ....20% to 22% by volume

Carbon dioxide...1,000 ppm maximum

Carbon monoxide ....20 ppm maximum

Total hydrocarbons other than methane ....25 ppm maximum

Particulates and oil mist...5 mg/m^3 maximum

Odor and taste ....Not objectionable

These standards are recognized as acceptable purity levels throughout the United States.

ARCHIMEDES PRINCIPLE AND GAS LAWS

Archimedes Principle: Any object wholly or partially immersed in a liquid is buoyed up by a force equal to the weight of the liquid displaced. (a) A negatively buoyant body sinks in a fluid because the weight of the fluid it displaces is less than the weight of the body. (b) A neutrally buoyant submerged body remains in equilibrium, neither rising nor sinking, because the weight of the fluid it displaces is exactly equal to its own weight. (c) A positively buoyant submerged body weighs less than the volume of liquid it displaces. It will rise and float with part of its volume above the surface. A floating body displaces its own weight of a liquid.

Boyle's Law: If the temperature is kept constant, the volume of a gas will vary inversely as the ABSOLUTE pressure while the density will vary directly as the pressure. Since the pressure and volume of a gas are inversely related—the higher the pressure, the smaller the volume, and vice-versa. The formula for Boyle's Law is:

$$PV = C$$

Where P = absolute pressure
V = volume
C = a constant

Charles' Law: If the pressure is kept constant, the volume of a gas will vary directly as the ABSOLUTE temperature. The amount of change in either volume or pressure is directly related to the change in absolute temperature. For example, if absolute temperature is doubled, then either the volume or the pressure also is doubled. The formula for Charles' Law is:

$$PV = RT \text{ or } \frac{PV = R}{T}$$

Where P = absolute pressure
V = volume
T = absolute temperature
R = a universal constant for all gases

General Gas Law: Boyle's Law illustrates pressure/volume relationships, and Charles' Law basically describes the effect of temperature changes on pressure and/or volume. The General Gas Law is a combination of these two laws. It is used to predict the behavior of a given quantity of gas when changes may be expected in any or all of the variables. The formula for the General Gas Law is:

$$\frac{P_1 V_1}{T_1} = \frac{P_2 V_2}{T_2}$$

Where P_1 = initial pressure (absolute)
V_1 = initial volume
T_1 = initial temperature (absolute)
P_2 = final pressure (absolute)
V_2 = final volume
T_2 = final temperature (absolute)

Dalton's Law: The total pressure exerted by a mixture of gases is equal to the sum of the pressures of each of the different gases making up the mixture—each gas acting as if it alone was present and occupied the total volume. The whole is equal to the sum of its parts and each part is not affected by any of the other parts. The pressure of any gas in the mixture is proportional to the number of molecules of that gas in the total volume. The pressure of each gas is called its partial pressure (pp), meaning its part of the whole. Dalton's Law is sometimes referred to as "the law of partial pressures." The formula for Dalton's Law is:

$$P_{Total} = PPA + PP_B + PP_C.....$$

and

$$PP_A = P_{Total} \times \frac{\%Vol._A}{100\%}$$

Where P_{Total} = Total absolute pressure of gas mixture
PP_A = Partial pressure of gas A
PP_B = Partial pressure of gas B
PP_C = Partial pressure of gas C

Henry's Law: The amount of a gas that will dissolve in a liquid at a given temperature is almost directly proportional to the partial pressure of that gas. If one unit of gas dissolves in a liquid at one atmosphere, then two units will dissolve at two atmospheres, three units at three atmospheres, etc.

AIR CONSUMPTION FORMULA/TABLE
(See p. 266)

Knowing your air consumption rate is very important. By determining your consumption rate at the surface, it becomes a simple matter to calculate what it will be at any given depth. Since pressure gauges are calibrated in pounds per square inch (psi), your consumption rate must be in psi too. The formula is as follows:

$$\frac{PSI \div TIME}{33/33 + DEPTH/33}$$

PSI = psi consumed in timed swim at a constant depth.
TIME = Duration of timed swim.
DEPTH = Depth of timed swim.

EXAMPLE:

A diver swims at a depth of 10 feet for 10 minutes and consumes 300 psi of air. You want to determine his surface consumption expressed in psi.

$$\frac{300\ (\text{PSI used})\ \div\ 10\ (\text{Time})\ =\ 30}{33/33\ +\ 10\ (\text{Depth})/33\ =\ 43/33} = \frac{30 \times 33}{43} = \frac{990}{43} = 23.02$$

23.02 PSI = PSI CONSUMED PER MINUTE AT SURFACE

NOTE: Consumption rate must be recalculated if tank size is changed. See table on p. 266.

SPORT DIVER OPEN WATER U.S. NAVY DIVE TABLES
(See illustration on p. 267)

COMPARISON OF SEVERAL POPULAR DIVE TABLES

Today, there are many dive tables available to the sport diver, derived from various theories and methodologies to determine the effect of saturated nitrogen, and all having the primary intent of assuring safety of the sport diver.

The new sport diver will learn from the dive table advocated by the agency providing the diving instruction.

Below is a synopsis of the no-decompression limits for air dives at various depths taken from 40 to 100 feet so that the reader can see the differences and similarities among the tables.

Maximum No-Decompression Limit

Depth	(1) U.S. Navy	(2) DCIEM	(3) PADI RDP	(4) PADI Wheel	(5) NAUI Table	(6) NAUI DTC 2
40	200	175	140	140	130	130
50	100	75	80	80	80	80
60	60	50	55	55	55	55
70	50	35	40	40	45	45
80	40	25	30	30	35	35
90	30	20	25	25	25	25
100	25	15	20	20	22	22

To clarify the sources of these figures, the following is provided as a reference to the above and relates to the numbers appearing above the respective column:

(1) U.S. Navy Air Decompression Table—Revision, May 1989.
(2) Sport Diving Tables—Department of National Defence (Canada) and produced under license by Universal Dive Tectronics, Inc., 2340 Vauxhall Place, Richmond, BC, Canada V6V 1YB–1987.
(3) Recreational Dive Planner—Diving Science & Technology Corp. and distributed by International PADI, Inc.
(4) The Wheel—Diving Science & Technology (DSAT) and distributed by International PADI, Inc., 1985, 1986, 1987, and 1988.

AIR CONSUMPTION TABLE AT DEPTH

DEPTH IN FEET

Surface	10	15	20	25	30	40	50	60	70	80	90	100	120	140	160
15	19.5	21.8	24.0	27.0	28.5	33.0	37.5	42.0	46.5	51	55.5	60	69	78	87
16	20.8	23.2	25.6	28.8	30.4	35.2	40.0	44.8	49.6	54.4	59.2	64	73.6	83.2	92.8
17	22.1	24.7	27.2	30.6	32.3	37.4	42.5	47.6	52.7	57.8	62.9	68	78.2	88.4	98.6
18	23.4	26.1	28.8	32.4	34.2	39.6	45.0	50.4	55.8	61.2	66.6	72	82.8	93.6	104.4
19	24.7	27.6	30.4	34.2	36.1	41.8	47.5	53.2	58.9	64.6	70.3	76	87.4	98.8	110.2
20	26.	29.0	32.0	36.0	38.0	44.0	50.0	56.0	62.0	68.0	74.0	80	92	104	116
21	27.3	30.5	33.6	37.8	39.9	46.2	52.5	58.8	65.1	71.4	77.7	84	96.6	109.2	121.8
22	28.6	31.9	35.2	39.6	41.8	48.4	55.0	61.6	68.2	74.8	81.4	88	101.2	114.4	127.6
23	29.9	33.4	36.8	41.4	43.7	50.6	57.5	64.4	71.3	78.2	85.1	92	105.8	119.6	133.4
24	31.2	34.8	38.4	43.2	45.6	52.8	60.	67.2	74.4	81.6	88.8	96	110.4	124.8	139.2
25	32.5	36.3	40.0	45.0	47.5	55.0	62.5	70.0	77.5	85.0	92.5	100	115	130	145
26	33.8	37.7	41.6	46.8	49.4	57.2	65.0	72.8	80.6	88.4	96.2	104	119.6	135.2	150.8
27	35.1	39.2	43.2	48.6	51.3	59.4	67.5	75.6	83.7	91.8	99.9	108	124.2	140.4	156.6
28	36.4	40.6	44.8	50.4	53.2	61.6	70.	78.4	86.8	95.2	103.6	112	128.8	145.6	162.4
29	37.7	42.1	46.4	52.2	55.1	63.8	72.5	81.2	89.9	98.6	107.3	116	133.4	150.8	168.2
30	39.	43.5	48.0	54.	57.0	66.0	75.0	84.0	93.0	102.0	111.0	120	138	156	174
31	40.3	45.0	49.6	55.8	58.9	68.2	77.5	86.8	96.1	105.4	114.7	124	142.6	161.2	179.8
32	41.6	46.4	51.2	57.6	60.8	70.4	80.0	89.6	99.2	108.8	118.4	128	147.2	166.4	185.6
33	42.9	47.9	52.8	59.4	62.7	72.6	82.5	92.4	102.3	112.2	122.1	132	151.8	171.6	191.4
34	44.2	49.3	54.4	61.2	64.6	74.8	85.0	95.2	105.4	115.6	125.8	136	156.4	176.8	197.2
35	45.5	50.8	56.0	63.0	66.5	77.0	87.5	98.0	108.5	119.0	129.5	140	161	182	203
36	46.8	52.2	57.6	64.8	68.4	79.2	90.0	100.8	111.6	122.4	133.2	144	165.6	187.2	208.8
37	48.1	53.7	59.2	66.6	70.3	81.4	92.5	103.6	114.7	125.8	136.9	148	170.2	192.4	214.6
38	49.4	55.1	60.8	68.4	72.2	83.6	95.0	106.4	117.8	129.2	140.6	152	174.8	197.6	220.4
39	50.7	56.6	62.4	70.2	74.1	85.8	97.5	109.2	120.9	132.6	144.3	156	179.4	202.8	226.2
40	52	58.	64.0	72.0	76.0	88.0	100.	112.0	124.0	136.	148.0	160	184	208	232

CONSUMPTION RATE AT SURFACE (PSI PER MINUTE)

no-decompression limits and repetitive group designation table for no-decompression air dives

Depth (feet)	No-decompression limits (min)	A	B	C	D	E	F	G	H	I	J	K	L	M	N	O
10		60	120	210	300											
15		35	70	110	160	225	350									
20		25	50	75	100	135	180	240	325							
25	(245)	20	35	55	75	100	125	160	195	245	315					
30	(205)	15	30	45	60	75	95	120	145	170	205	250	310			
35	(160) 310	5	15	25	40	50	60	80	100	120	140	160	190	220	270	310
40	(130) 200	5	15	25	30	40	50	70	80	100	110	130	150	170	200	
50	(70) 100		10	15	25	30	40	50	60	70	80	90	100			
60	(50) 60		10	15	20	25	30	40	50	55	60					
70	(40) 50		5	10	15	20	30	35	40	45	50					
80	(30) 40		5	10	15	20	25	30	35	40						
90	(25) 30		5	10	12	15	20	25	30							
100	(20) 25		5	7	10	15	20	22	25							
110	(15) 20			5	10	13	15	20								
120	(10) 15			5	10	12	15									
130	(5) 10			5	8	10										
140	10			5	7	10										

residual nitrogen timetable for repetitive air dives

*Dives following surface intervals of more than 12 hours are not repetitive dives. Use actual bottom times in the Standard Air Decompression Tables to compute decompression for such dives.

The red line and red numbers on the no-decompression limits table above provide recommended limits based on ultrasound studies. The U.S. Navy Dive Table limits are based on extremely physically fit young males. For added safety, stop at 10 feet for one to three minutes at the end of each no-decompression dive. This helps to deplete most or all small nitrogen bubbles.

The black line on the lower table denotes U.S. Navy no-decompression limits. All residual nitrogen times listed to the left of the line will require the use of the Standard Air Decompression Table to compute decompression times and depths.

Repetitive group at the beginning of the surface interval

Surface interval time ranges (read resulting **NEW GROUP** from the column headers):

Repetitive group at beginning	Z	O	N	M	L	K	J	I	H	G	F	E	D	C	B	A
A																0:10–12:00*
B															0:10–2:10	2:11–12:00*
C														0:10–1:39	1:40–2:49	2:50–12:00*
D													0:10–1:09	1:10–2:38	2:39–5:48	5:49–12:00*
E												0:10–0:54	0:55–1:57	1:58–3:22	3:23–6:32	6:33–12:00*
F											0:10–0:45	0:46–1:29	1:30–2:28	2:29–3:57	3:58–7:05	7:06–12:00*
G										0:10–0:40	0:41–1:15	1:16–1:59	2:00–2:58	2:59–4:25	4:26–7:35	7:36–12:00*
H									0:10–0:36	0:37–1:06	1:07–1:41	1:42–2:23	2:24–3:20	3:21–4:49	4:50–7:59	8:00–12:00*
I								0:10–0:33	0:34–0:59	1:00–1:29	1:30–2:02	2:03–2:44	2:45–3:43	3:44–5:12	5:13–8:21	8:22–12:00*
J							0:10–0:31	0:32–0:54	0:55–1:19	1:20–1:47	1:48–2:20	2:21–3:04	3:05–4:02	4:03–5:40	5:41–8:40	8:41–12:00*
K						0:10–0:28	0:29–0:49	0:50–1:11	1:12–1:35	1:36–2:03	2:04–2:38	2:39–3:21	3:22–4:19	4:20–5:48	5:49–8:58	8:59–12:00*
L					0:10–0:26	0:27–0:45	0:46–1:04	1:05–1:25	1:26–1:49	1:50–2:19	2:20–2:53	2:54–3:36	3:37–4:35	4:36–6:02	6:03–9:12	9:13–12:00*
M				0:10–0:25	0:26–0:42	0:43–0:59	1:00–1:18	1:19–1:39	1:40–2:05	2:06–2:34	2:35–3:08	3:09–3:52	3:53–4:49	4:50–6:18	6:19–9:28	9:29–12:00*
N			0:10–0:24	0:25–0:39	0:40–0:54	0:55–1:11	1:12–1:30	1:31–1:53	1:54–2:18	2:19–2:47	2:48–3:22	3:23–4:04	4:05–5:03	5:04–6:32	6:33–9:43	9:44–12:00*
O		0:10–0:23	0:24–0:36	0:37–0:51	0:52–1:07	1:08–1:24	1:25–1:43	1:44–2:04	2:05–2:29	2:30–2:59	3:00–3:33	3:34–4:17	4:18–5:16	5:17–6:44	6:45–9:54	9:55–12:00*
Z	0:10–0:22	0:23–0:34	0:35–0:48	0:49–1:02	1:03–1:18	1:19–1:36	1:37–1:55	1:56–2:17	2:18–2:42	2:43–3:10	3:11–3:45	3:46–4:29	4:30–5:27	5:28–6:56	6:57–10:05	10:06–12:00*

NEW GROUP DESIGNATION →	Z	O	N	M	L	K	J	I	H	G	F	E	D	C	B	A
REPETITIVE DIVE DEPTH																
40	257	241	213	187	161	138	116	101	87	73	61	49	37	25	17	7
50	169	160	142	124	111	99	87	76	66	56	47	38	29	21	13	6
60	122	117	107	97	88	79	70	61	52	44	36	30	24	17	11	5
70	100	96	87	80	72	64	57	50	43	37	31	26	20	15	9	4
80	84	80	73	68	61	54	48	43	38	32	28	23	18	13	8	4
90	73	70	64	58	53	47	43	38	33	29	24	20	16	11	7	3
100	64	62	57	52	48	43	38	34	30	26	22	18	14	10	7	3
110	57	55	51	47	42	38	34	31	27	24	20	16	13	10	6	3
120	52	50	46	43	39	35	32	28	25	21	18	15	12	9	6	3
130	46	44	40	38	35	31	28	25	22	19	16	13	11	8	6	3
140	42	40	38	35	32	29	26	23	20	18	15	12	10	7	5	2

residual nitrogen times (minutes)

JEPPESEN

(5) Dive Tables—National Association of Underwater Instructors, 1990.

(6) Dive Time Calculator II—National Association of Underwater Instructors, 1989.

To take this analysis further, we will assume that a dive team makes a dive to 60 feet for 40 minutes. The divers then return to the surface and have a surface interval time (SIT) of 3 hours, 20 minutes, following which the divers perform a second dive to 40 feet for 60 minutes. We compare how the divers are treated by each of the above tables relative to Repetitive Dive Group after dive No. 1, Residual Nitrogen Times if applicable, Dive Group at the beginning of the second dive, Maximum allowable bottom time on the second dive, and Repetitive Dive Group after dive No. 2.

Repetitive Dive Group* at the end of dive 1

	U.S. Navy	DCIEM	PADI RDP	PADI Wheel	NAUI Table	NAUI DTC 2
60 feet for 40 min	G	E	Q	Q	G	G

Residual Nitrogen at beginning of dive 2 after SIT

Depth	U.S. Navy	DCIEM	PADI RDP	PADI Wheel	NAUI Table	NAUI DTC 2
40 feet	25	40†	9	‡	25	25

Group Designation at beginning of dive 2

	U.S. Navy	DCIEM	PADI RDP	PADI Wheel	NAUI TABLE	NAUI DTC 2
3:20 SIT	B	N/A	A	A	C	C

Though the dive plan calls for a second dive for 60 minutes, the maximum adjusted no-decompression limit for the second dive is as follows:

Depth	U.S. Navy	DCIEM	PADI RDP	PADI Wheel	NAUI Table	NAUI DTC 2
40 feet	175	135	131	131	105	105

Group designation at the end of dive 2

Depth	U.S. Navy	DCIEM	PADI RDP	PADI Wheel	NAUI Table	NAUI DTC 2
40 feet for 60 min	I	N/A	P	P	I	I

NOTE: Group designation is indicated N/A under the DCIEM table due to the unique way that repetitive dives are computed using their table.

---

*The Wheel and Recreational Dive Planner use the term pressure group (PG) rather than repetitive dive group and cannot be used to enter any table using the repetitive dive group designations, as the groupings are based on the research and theories of DSAT only. Users of the Wheel and the Recreational Dive Planner may use either interchangeably, as they are based on the same research and theories.

†Due to the methodology used by the DCIEM tables, this is an interpolated value.

‡The Wheel does not give residual nitrogen times.

Unit	Abbreviation	Number of	Approximate U.S. equivalent		
Length					
myriameter	mym	10,000 meters	6.2 miles		
kilometer	km	1,000 meters	0.62 mile		
hectometer	hm	100 meters	109.36 yards		
dekameter	dam	10 meters	32.81 feet		
meter	m	1 meters	39.37 inches		
decimeter	dm	0.1 meters	3.94 inches		
centimeter	cm	0.01 meters	0.39 inch		
millimeter	mm	0.001 meters	0.04 inch		
Area					
square kilometer	sq km or km^2	1,000,000 sq. meters	0.3861 square mile		
hectare	ha	10,000 sq. meters	2.47 acres		
arc	a	100 sq. meters	119.60 square yards		
centare	ca	1 sq. meters	10.76 square feet		
square centimeter	sq cm or cm^2	0.0001 sq. meters	0.155 square inch		
Volume					
dekastere	das	10 cubic meters	13.10 cubic yards		
stere	s	1 cubic meters	1.31 cubic yards		
decistere	ds	0.10 cubic meters	3.53 cubic feet		
cubic centimeter	cu cm or cm' also cc	0.000001 cubic meters	0.061 cubic inch		
Capacity			CUBIC	DRY	LIQUID
kiloliter	kl	1,000 liters	1.31 cubic yards		
hectoliter	hl	100 liters	3.53 cubic feet	2.84 bushels	
dekaliter	dal	10 liters	0.35 cubic foot	1.14 pecks	2.64 gallons
liter	l	1 liters	61.02 cubic inches	0.908 quart	1.057 quarts
deciliter	dl	0.10 liters	6.1 cubic inches	0.18 pint	0.21 pint
centiliter	cl	0.01 liters	0.6 cubic inch		0.338 fluidounce
milliliter	ml	0.001 liters	0.06 cubic inch		0.27 fluidram

CONVERSION FACTORS

To convert			Multiply by
Length			
cm	to	inches	0.394
meters		feet	3.28
kilometers		nautical miles	0.540
inches	to	cm	2.54
feet		meters	0.3048
nautical miles		kilometers	1.853
Area			
cm^2	to	inches^2	0.155
meters^2		feet^2	10.76
kilometers^2		miles^2	0.386
inches^2	to	cm^2	6.45
feet^2		meters^2	0.093
miles^2		kilometers^2	0.3861
Volume and Capacity			
cc or ml	to	cu. inches	0.061
cu. meters		cu. feet	35.31
liters		cu. inches	61.02
liters		cu. feet	0.035
liters		fluid oz	33.81
liters		quarts	1.057
cu. inches	to	cc or ml	16.39
cu. feet		cu. meters	0.0283
quarts		liters	0.946
Weight			
grams	to	ounces	0.035
kilograms		pounds	2.205
ounces	to	grams	28.35
pounds		kilograms	0.454
Temperature			
°C	to	°F	9/5 then add 32
°F		°C	5/9 after subtracting 32
Pressure			
pounds per sq. in.	to	kg/cm^2	0.0703
pounds per sq. in.		cm of Hg	5.17
pounds per sq. in.		ft. of seawater	2.18
feet of seawater		psi	0.445

U.S. WEIGHTS AND MEASURES

Unit	Abbreviation or symbol	U.S. equivalent	Approximate metric equivalent
Length			
mile	mi	5280 feet, 320 rods, 1760 yards	1,609 kilometers
rod	rd	5.50 yards, 16.5 feet	5.029 meters
yard	yd	3 feet, 36 inches	0.914 meters
foot	ft or '	12 inches, 0.333 yards	30.480 centimeters
inch	in or "	0.083 feet, 0.027 yards	2.540 centimeters
Area			
square mile	sq mi or mi^2	640 acres, 102,400 square rods	2,590 square kilometers
acre		4840 square yards, 43,560 square feet	0.405 hectares, 4047 square meters
square rod	sq rd or rd^2	30.25 square yards, 0.006 acres	25.293 square meters
square yard	sq yd or yd^2	1296 square inches, 9 square feet	0.836 square meters
square foot	sq ft or ft^2	144 square inches, 0.111 square yards	0.093 square meters
square inch	sq in or in^2	0.007 square feet, 0.00077 square yards	6.451 square centimeters
Volume			
cubic yard	cu yd or yd^3	27 cubic feet, 46,656 cubic inches	0.765 cubic meters
cubic foot	cu ft or ft^3	1728 cubic inches, 0.0370 cubic yards	0.028 cubic meters
cubic inch	cu in or in^3	0.00058 cubic feet, 0.000021 cubic yards	16.387 cubic centimeters
Capacity			
		U.S. liquid measure	
gallon	gal	4 quarts (231 cubic inches)	3.785 liters
quart	qt	2 pints (57.75 cubic inches)	0.946 liters
pint	pt	4 gills (28.875 cubic inches)	0.473 liters
gill	gi	4 fluidounces (7.218 cubic inches)	118.291 milliliters
fluidounce	fl oz	8 fluidrams (1.804 cubic inches)	29.573 milliliters
fluidram	fl dr	60 minims (0.225 cubic inches)	3.696 milliliters
minim	min	1/00 fluidram (0.003759 cubic inches)	0.061610 milliliters

Continued.

U.S. WEIGHTS AND MEASURES—cont'd

Unit	Abbreviation or symbol	U.S. equivalent	Approximate metric equivalent
Weight			
		Avoirdupois	
ton		20 short hundred-	
short ton		weight, 2000 pounds	0.907 metric tons
long ton		20 long hundredweight, 2240 pounds	1.016 metric tons
hundredweight	cwt		
short hundredweight		100 pounds, 0.05 short tons	45.159 kilograms
long hundredweight		112 pounds, 0.05 long tons	50.802 kilograms
pound	lb	16 ounces, 7000 grains	0.453 kilograms
ounce	ox	16 drams, 437.5 grains	28.349 grams
dram	dr	27.343 grains, 0.0625 ounces	1.771 grams
grain	gr	0.036 drams, 0.002285 ounces	0.0648 grams
		Troy	
pound	lb t	12 ounces, 240 penny-weight, 5760 grains	0.373 kilograms
ounce	oz t	20 pennyweight, 480 grains	31.103 grams
pennyweight	dwt also pwt	24 grains, 0.05 ounces	1.555 grams
grain	gr	0.042 pennyweight, 0.002083 ounces	0.0648 grams

LOCATING YOUR NEAREST RECOMPRESSION CHAMBER

The following numbers may be called 24 hours a day, 7 days a week. Physicians are on call and consultation can be provided on air embolism or decompression sickness cases. Each maintains a world-wide listing of recompression chambers.

Divers Alert Network
DAN
919-684-8111

U.S. Navy Experimental Diving Unit
EDU Duty Phone
904-234-4353

EQUIPMENT CHECK LIST

Diving equipment

_____ Swim suit
_____ Mask
_____ Snorkel and snorkel keeper
_____ Fins
_____ Wet or dry suit
_____ Jacket
_____ Booties
_____ Gloves
_____ Pants
_____ Vest
_____ Hood
_____ Weight belt and weights
_____ Buoyancy compensator
_____ Full tank
_____ Regulator
_____ SPG
_____ Watch
_____ Depth gauge
_____ Compass
_____ Decompression tables
_____ Diver's flag and float
_____ Ascent/descent line and weight
_____ Whistle
_____ Knife
_____ Logbook and pencils
_____ Gear bag

Specialty items

_____ Diving computer
_____ Thermometer
_____ Emergency flare
_____ Dive light and batteries
_____ Slate and pencil
_____ Safety line (200 feet minimum)
_____ Buddy line
_____ Alternate air source

_____ Lift bag
_____ Photography equipment
_____ Strobe
_____ Camera
_____ Film
_____ Housing
_____ Batteries
_____ Spearfishing gear
_____ Speargun
_____ Game bag
_____ Fishing license

Spare parts and repair kit

_____ Mask strap and buckle
_____ Fin strap and buckle
_____ "O" rings
_____ Regulator high-pressure plug
_____ Silicone spray/grease
_____ Wet suit cement
_____ Sewing repair kit
_____ Extra mask lens
_____ Waterproof plastic tape
_____ Pliers/wrench/diver's tool
_____ Small knife
_____ BC repair patches

_____ **Other items**

_____ Dry clothes
_____ Towels
_____ Food and drinking water
_____ Sunglasses
_____ Suntan lotion
_____ Logbook
_____ Certification card
_____ Marine life identification guide

FIRST AID KIT COMPONENTS

_____ Utility shears
_____ Pocket mask with case
_____ Small flashlight with batteries
_____ Malleable, reusable splint
_____ 3-, 4-, and 6-inch conforming bandage
_____ 4 × 4 inch dressings
_____ Multitrauma dressing
_____ Triangular bandages
_____ 3 inch hypoallergenic tape
_____ 1 inch BandAids
_____ Burn dressings
_____ Cold packs
_____ Hot packs
_____ Disposable blanket for hypothermia
_____ Oral glucose

_____ Sterile sodium chloride solution (1 L minimum)
_____ Isopropyl alcohol
_____ Ammonia solution
_____ Acetic acid solution
_____ Antibiotic ointment
_____ Corticosteroid anti-inflammatory ointment
_____ Oral diphenhydramine (Benadryl)
_____ Nonaspirin pain reliever
_____ Aspirin
_____ Motion sickness medication
_____ Sunblocker
_____ Shaving cream
_____ Disposable razors
_____ Cleansing towelettes

Index

A

Abalone, 229
Absolute pressure, 132
Accessories, 92-101
Accident, prevention of, 145-149
Acid rain, 226
Aids to dive planning, 168-170
Air
    alternate sources of, 67
    clean, 129, 130
Air consumption, formula/tables for, 264, 265
Air embolism, 142-144
    first aid for, 143, 144
Air masses, 176
Air pressure, 132-135
Air purity standards, 263
Alcohol, 151
Alga, 197
Allergic reaction, 140
Altitude, high, diving in, 132, 158, 189
Aluminum 80, 55
Aluminum tank, 61
Alveoli, 117, 118
Ambient pressure, 64, 132
American Academy of Underwater Sciences, 260
Amphibians, fresh water, 216
Anemone, 202
Angel fish, 200-202
Animals
    fresh water, 215-217
    marine, dangerous, 205-207
    underwater, 196
Anxiety, 151
Archimedes principle, 263, 264
Ascending, 32
    and descending, 131-149
Ascent
    emergency, 146-149
    procedures for, 145-149
    rate of, 156, 157
Asphyxia, 124
Atmosphere of pressure, 132

B

Back roll entry, 25
Backpack, 59, 60

Backrush, 186, 187
Barometer, 177
Barracuda, 205, 206
BC; see Buoyancy compensator
Belt; see Weight belt
Bends; see Decompression sickness
Bezel, 83
Birth control pills, 235
    decompression sickness and, 156
Blackout, shallow water, 122
Blade design of fins, 14
Blasting of regulator, 73
Blue-water diving, 254, 255
Boat, entries from, 24-27
Boat divers, effects of currents on, 192-194
Body temperature, maintaining, 108, 113, 114
Boot(s), 37-39
    for tanks, 59
Booties, 15
Bottom formation in cold water, 199
Bottom time, 157, 158
    defined, 164
Bourdon tube depth gauge, 85
Boyle's law, 137-138, 263
Breath, holding of, 145
Breathing, 116-130
    buddy, 75-77
    skip, 122
Breathing resistance, 64
Breathing rhythm, 121
Breathing underwater, 51-79
    history of, 52-54
Bronchi, 117, 118
Bubbles, nitrogen, 154, 155, 162
Buckle(s), 39, 40
    weight belt, 44
Buddy breathing, 75-77
Buddy system, 78, 79
Buoyancy, 32, 43, 102-104
    changes in, 103, 104
    control of, 102, 103
    entry and, 24
    of fins, 14
    and warmth, 33-50
    wet suit material and, 35
Buoyancy compensator (BC), 46-50
    care and maintenance of, 49, 50
    selection of, 46-48
    use of, 39, 48, 49

C

Caisson disease, 154
Canadian Transport Commission (CTC), 56
Capillaries, 117, 118
Capillary gauge, 84
Carbon dioxide, 151
    respiration and, 121, 122
Cardiopulmonary resuscitation (CPR),
    125-129
Careers, 256-261
Cave(s), 213, 214
    characteristics of, 248
    types of, 246-248
Cave diving, 246-249
Cavern diving, 250, 251
Chamber, recompression; *see* Recompression
    chamber
Charles' law, 263
Chart, water temperature protection, 262
Checklist for equipment, 273
Chemical dumping, 223
Chemical glow light, 95
Chokes, 154
Clams, 230
Clean air, 129, 130
Clearing of mask, 11
CO₂ cartridge, 47, 49
Coastal problems, 221-225
Cold water(s), 34, 35, 37
    bottom formation in, 199
    effects of, 114
Color, seeing underwater and, 106
Commercial development of sea for food, 232
Commercial fishing, ecology and, 224
Commercial work in diving, 259, 260
Compass, 87-90
Conch, 230
Conditioning, diving and, 234-236
Conduction, body temperature and, 113, 114
Construction, ecology and, 222, 223
Contact lenses, 9
Contamination of air, 129, 130
Continental shelf, 172, 173
Conversion of feet to meters of seawater,
    85
Conversion factors, 270
Coral(s), 196-198
    fire, 207
    water temperature and, 199

Coral reef entries, 189
Corrosion, 56
CPR; *see* Cardiopulmonary resuscitation
Crab, 204, 231
Crustaceans, 204, 230, 231
CTC; *see* Canadian Transport Commission
Current(s)
    boat divers and, 192-194
    localized, 190-194
    tidal, 181-183

D

Dalton's law, 264
Damage, oil, 223, 224
Dangerous marine animals, 205-207
DCS; *see* Decompression sickness
Decompression diving, 168
Decompression stage, 154
Decompression sickness (DCS), 86, 153-160
    prevention of, 155, 156
    symptoms of, 155
    treatment of, 159, 160
Decreasing pressure, 142-144
Deflation, 48
Defoggers, 10
Defogging solution, 10
Demand regulator; *see* Regulator
Depth
    defined, 164
    reef formation and, 198, 199
Depth gauge, 83-85
Depth limits, 150-160
Descending and ascending, 131-149
Devices, pressure, time, and direction, 81-90
Dewpoint, 177
Diaphragm, 117-119
Diaphragm depth gauge, 85
Diet, diving and, 140, 141, 234, 235
DIN connection, 58
Direction devices, 81-90
Disc, frangible, 58
Ditching, 147
    of weight belt, 45, 46
Dive(s)
    repetitive, 161-170
    surface, 30-32
Dive computers, 86, 87

Dive conditions, predicting, 240, 241
Dive day, planning and, 240
Dive flag, 93
Dive knife, 95, 96
Dive planning; *see* Planning
Dive profile, 164-168
Dive skins, 34
Dive tables, 86, 87, 97-99, 265-268
Dive tool, 95, 96
Divers, women, 235, 236
Divers Alert Network (DAN), 237, 272
    air embolism and, 144
    recompression and, 160
Diving
    specialty, 245-256
    on the water planet, 178
    worlds of, 171-178
Diving areas, fresh water, 209-215
Diving watch, 83
Dock, entries from, 24-27
Dolphin kick, 18
DOT; *see* U.S. Department of Transportation
Drowning, 123
    first aid for, 124, 125
Drugs, diving and, 140, 141
Dry suit, 41, 42, 141
Dump valve, 47
Dumping, chemical, 223

E

Ear discomfort, 12
Ear squeeze, 138-140
Earplugs, 141
Ecology, 173, 218-226
    coastal problems and, 221-225
    industry and, 223, 224
    inland problems and, 225, 226
    solutions and, 226
    sources of problems and, 219-221
    sport diving and, 224, 225
Eel, 206
Effects of pressure change, 132-136
Electronic depth gauge, 85
Embolism; *see* Air embolism
Emergency ascent, 146-149
Emphysema, 144
Entries, 23-30, 187-189

Environmental considerations, 239
Environmental variation, 173-178
Equalization, 8, 12, 139, 140
Equipment checklist, 273
Equipment preparation, 238, 239
Equipment squeezes, 141
Eutrophication, 226
Evaporation, body temperature and, 113, 114
Examination, physical, 145, 234
Exhaustion, 123, 124
Exposure, 108, 113-115

F

Farmer Johns, 35
Fatigue, 151
Fear, 123
Featherduster worms, 202
Fins, 12-20
    blade design of, 14
    fit of, 14, 15
    selection of, 13-15
    use of, 39
Fire coral, 207
First aid
    for air embolism, 143, 144
    for drowning, 124, 125
First aid kit, 237, 238, 274
First stage, 64, 65
First stage reserves, 67-69
Fish
    fresh water, 215, 216
    tropical, 200-202
Fishing, commercial, ecology and, 224
Fit
    of fins, 14, 15
    of wet suit, 37
Flag and float, 93, 94
Flare, 95
Float and flag, 93, 94
Floating, 102
Flutter kick, 17
Flying after diving, 159
Fog, 177
Food
    commercial development of sea for, 232
    from sea and lake, 227-232
Footwear, 12-20

Forecasting of weather, 177, 178, 239, 240
Frangible disc, 58
Frenzel maneuver, 12
Fresh water, 208-217
    animals of, 215-217
    diving areas in, 209-215
Freshwater entries, 189
Frog kick, 18
Fronts, 176, 177

G

Garbage, 221, 222
Gas exchange, 120-123
Gas laws, 263, 264
Gauge; *see also* Submersible pressure gauge
    capillary, 84
    depth, 83-85
    pressure, 132
Gear bag, 100
Glass in lens of mask, 6
Glasses, prescription, 9
Gloves, use of, 40
Goggles, 5, 141
Golden triangle concept, 67

H

Hand signals, 108-113
Hangover, 151
Hawaiian sling, 228, 229
Headache, respiration and, 121, 122
Hearing, underwater, 107, 108
Henry's law, 154, 264
History
    of breathing underwater, 52-54
    of ocean, 172, 173
Holding of breath, 145
Hood(s), 141
    use of, 39
Horse collar, 46, 47
Hungry for air, 121, 122
Hydrostatic testing, 63
Hyperventilation, 122, 123
Hypothermia, 114
Hypoxia, 122

I

Ice diving, 251, 252
Industry, ecology and, 223, 224
Inexperience, 151
Infection, diving and, 140
Inflation, oral, 48
Inflation device, 47
Inflator, 47
Inhabitants of reef, 200-204
Inland problems and ecology, 225, 226
Inspection of scuba tanks, 61-63
Instruction, careers in, 257, 258
International Diving Education Association
    (IDEA), 257
Intestine squeeze, 141
Invertebrates, 202-203

J

J valve, 57, 68
Jacket(s)
    use of, 39
    wet suit, 37
Journalism, sport diving careers and, 258, 259

K

K valve, 57
Kelp, 199
Kicking, 17-20

L

Lakes, 210, 211
    food from, 227-232
Law(s)
    Boyle's, 137-138
    gas, 263, 264
    Henry's, 154
    Martini's, 151
Legal rights to items found, 253
Lens(es)
    contact, 9
    of masks, 6

Life
  marine, handling of, 207
  ocean, 195-207
Light
  chemical glow, 95
  seeing underwater and, 104
  underwater, 96, 97
Limnology, 261
Lining of wet suits, 36
Lobster, 204, 231
Logbook, 97-99
Longshore currents, 190
Los Angeles County Underwater Instructors
      Association, 257
Lubber line, 88
Lubricants, 130
Lung(s), 117-119, 144
Lung squeeze, 141
Lung volumes, 119, 120

M

Mammals, fresh water, 217
Manatee, 217
Marine animals, dangerous, 205-207
Marine life, handling of, 207
Markings on scuba tanks, 56, 57
Martini's law, 151
Mask(s), 4-12
  clearing of, 11
  features of, 8, 9
  fit of, 9
  seeing with, 104
  selection of, 6, 7
  use of, 10-12, 40
Mask squeeze, 12, 141
Measures and weights, 271, 272
Mediastinal emphysema, 144
Medication, diving and, 140, 141
Menstrual periods, 235, 236
Metric system, 269
Mines, 215
Moray eel, 206
Mouth to mouth resuscitation, 125-129
Mouthpiece for snorkel, 21, 22
Movement of water, 179-184
Multinational Diving Education Association,
      257

N

Narcosis, nitrogen, 151, 152
Narcotic effects of nitrogen, 151
National Association for Cave Diving (NACD),
      213, 249
National Association for Search and Rescue
      (NASAR), 255
National Association of Underwater Instructors
      (NAUI), 258
National Association of Scuba Diving Schools
      (NASDS), 257
National Ocean Service (NOS), 183
National Oceanic and Atmospheric Adminis-
      tration (NOAA), 177
National Speleological Society—Cave Diving
      Section (NSS-CDS), 213, 249
National YMCA Scuba Program, 258
Natural navigation, 90, 91
Navigation, natural, 90, 91
Neoprene, 35
Nitrogen; *see also* Residual nitrogen
  respiration and, 120, 121
Nitrogen bubbles, 154, 155, 162
Nitrogen narcosis, 151, 152
No-decompression limit, 265-267
  table for, 156, 157
Nutrition, diving and, 234, 235

O

"O" ring, 57
Obesity, decompression sickness and,
      156
Objectives of dive, 236
Ocean life, 195-207
Oceanography, 260, 261
Octocorallia, 197
Octopus regulator, 66, 76
Oil damage, 223, 224
Oral inflation, 48
Overpressure injuries, 144
Overturns, 175, 176
Oxidation, 56
Oxygen
  respiration and, 121, 122
  tolerance for, 152
Oxygen system, planning and, 237, 238

Oxygen toxicity, 153
Oysters, 230

P

Panic, 123, 124
Pants, 37
Parrotfish, 200
Partial pressure, 152, 153
Photography, sport diving careers and, 259
Physical examination, 145, 234
Phytoplankton, 174
Pike, 216
Planning, 233-244
    aids to, 168-170
    conditioning and, 234-236
    dive day and, 240
    equipment preparation and, 238, 239
    objectives and, 236
    site selection and scouting and, 236, 237
    weather forecasting and, 239, 240
Pneumopericardium, 144
Pneumothorax, 144
Pockets, wet suit, 37
Pollution, 221, 222
Pool deck, entries from, 24-27
Porgies, 200
Predicting the dive conditions, 240, 241
Pregnancy, 235
    decompression sickness and, 156
Preparation of equipment, 238, 239
Prescription glasses, 9
Pressure
    air, 132-135
    ambient, 64
    change of, 132-136
    decreasing, 142-144
    depth and time limits and, 151
    increasing, 136-142
    in middle ears and sinuses, 8
    partial, 152, 153
    tank, 64, 65
    water, 132-135
Pressure devices, 81-90
Pressure squeeze, 136
Prevention
    of decompression sickness, 155, 156
    of diving accidents, 145-149

Prevention—cont'd
    of nitrogen narcosis, 151, 152
Professional Association of Diving Instructors
        (PADI), 258
Professional Diving Instructors Corporation
        (PDIC), 258
Purge valve, 8, 11
Purging of regulator, 73

Q

Quarries, 212, 213

R

R valve, 68
Rate of ascent, 156, 157
Reciprocal dive courses, 89
Recompression, underwater, 160
Recompression chamber, 159
    locating, 272
Recovery of regulator, 75
Recreational Scuba Training Council (RCTS),
        145
Reef(s), 186
    development of, 196-198
    formation and depths and, 198, 199
    inhabitants of, 200-204
Refraction, 4, 104, 105
Regulator, 63-75
    assembly of, 70-72
    clearing of, 73
    disassembly, care, and maintenance of, 72
    lubricants for, 130
    octopus, 66, 76
    recovery of, 75
    selection of, 64-68
    use of, 69
Repair kit, 99
Repetitive dive(s), 161-170
    defined, 164
    typical, 162-164
Reptiles, fresh water, 217
Rescue; *see* Search and rescue
Reserve, options for, 66-69
Residual nitrogen, 162-168
Respiration, 117-123

Respiratory system, 117-119
Resuscitation, 125-129
Rhythm, breathing, 121
Rip currents, 190-192
Rivers, 211, 212
Rock, 199
Rocky shore entries, 189
Rounding in use of tables, 158

S

Safety, 243, 244
 ice diving and, 252
Safety stop, 146
Sand beach entries, 187-189
Sandbar, 186
Sandpits, 212, 213
Scallops, 230
Sciences, careers and, 260, 261
Scissors kick, 18
Scleractinia, 197
Scouting of dive site, 236, 237
Scuba Schools International, 258
Scuba tank(s), 54-63
 aluminum, warning about, 56
 boots for, 59
 care and maintenance of, 60, 61
 cleaning of, 62, 63
 coatings for, 56
 hydrostatic testing of, 63
 markings for, 56, 57
 selection of, 55-60
 steel, 56
 visual inspection of, 61-63
Sea, food from, 227-232
Sea urchin, 202
Search and rescue (SAR), 255
Second stage, 65
Seeing, 104-106
 and swimming, 3-32
Sensations, 101-115
Seventy-two tank, 55
Sewage, 221, 222
Shallow water blackout, 122
Shark, 205
Shellfish, 229, 230
Shivering, 114
Shore entries, 27-30

Shrimp, 232
Signals, hand, 108-113
Sinkholes, 215, 248
Sinus squeeze, 140, 141
Siphon, 248
Site selection, 236
Skip breathing, 122
Skirt of mask, 9
Slack time, 181
Slack water, 181
Slate, 98
Snorkel, 20-23
 breathing and, 121
 use of, 22, 23
Socks, 37, 39
Solution, defogging, 10
Sound, underwater, 107, 108
Sources of air, alternate, 67
Spare parts, 99
Speaking, underwater, 107, 108
Spearfishing, 228, 229
Speargun, 229
Specialty diving, 245-256
SPG; *see* Submersible pressure gauge
Sport diver, standards for safe diving of, 243, 244
Sport diving
 careers in, 257-259
 ecology and, 224, 225
Springs, 215, 248
Squeeze(s), 138-142
 mask, 12
 pressure, 136
Squirrel fish, 200
Stage decompression, 154
Standards
 air purity, 263
 for safe diving, 243, 244
Starfish, 202
Sting ray, 206, 207
Stomach squeeze, 141
Stop, safety, 146
Strap
 lens, 7
 mask, 10
Submersible pressure gauge (SPG), 68, 69, 81, 82
Sunburn, 115
Sunfish, 215
Surf, formation of, 185-187
Surf zone, 186

Surface dives, 30-32
Surface interval time, 164
Surfacing, 32
Surge, 189, 190
Swimming, seeing and, 3-32
Symbiosis, 220
Symptoms
    of decompression sickness, 155
    of nitrogen narcosis, 151, 152

T

Table(s)
    air consumption, 264, 265
    dive, 86, 87, 97-99, 265-268
    rounding in use of, 158
    selection of, 157
    tidal current, 183
Tank(s); *see* Scuba tank(s)
Temperature
    body, maintaining, 108, 113, 114
    of water, 34, 35, 173-176
Tempered safety glass for lens, 6
Testing, hydrostatic, 63
Thermoclines, 175
Thermometer, 97
Tidal volume, 119, 120
Tide(s), 180, 181
Time
    bottom, 157, 158
    slack, 181
Time devices, 81-90
Time limits, 150-160
Timing devices, underwater, 82, 83
Tolerance for oxygen, 152
Tool(s), 92-101
Tooth squeeze, 142
Trachea, 117, 118
Training, cave diving and, 249
Trapeze, 255
Treasure hunting, 253, 254
Turbidity, seeing and, 106

U

Undertow, 186, 187
Underwater animals, 196

Underwater breathing, 51-79
Underwater light, 96, 97
Underwater recompression, 160
Uprush, 186, 187
Upwellings, 176
U.S. Coast Guard Auxiliary, 181
U.S. Department of Transportation (DOT), 56
U.S. Navy standard air decompression tables, 156, 157
U.S. Navy Experimental Diving Unit, 272
U.S. Power Squadron, 181
U.S. weights and measures, 271, 272

V

Valve(s), 68
    dump, 47
    purge, 8, 11
    tank, 57-59
Variation, environmental, 173-178
Vented-blade fins, 14
Vertigo, 142
Visibility, 240-242

W

Warning about tanks, 56
Warmth
    and buoyancy, 33-50
    maintaining, 114
Water
    fresh; *see* Fresh water
    slack, 181
Water movement, 179-194
Water pressure, 132-135
Water temperature, 34, 35, 173-176
Water temperature protection chart, 262
Waves, 183-190
Weather, 176-178
    forecasting of, 177, 178, 239, 240
Weight belt, 39, 40, 42-46
    ditching of, 147
    selecting of, 42-45
    use of, 45, 46
Weights and measures, 271, 272
Wet suit, 37-41
    care and maintenance of, 41

Wet suit—cont'd
    features of, 36, 37
    fit of, 37
    selection of, 35, 36
    use of, 37-40
Whistle, 94
Wind, 241
Wind waves, 183-185
Windpipe, 117, 118
Women divers, 235, 236

Work, commercial, in diving, 259, 260
Worlds of diving, 171-178
Worms, 202
Wreck diving, 252, 253

Z

Zippers in boots, 39

Just Add Water

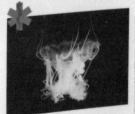

Jeppesen's ADVANCED SPORT DIVER MANUAL
2nd Edition

Richard A. Clinchy, III, Glen Egstrom, and Lou Fead
December 1992   ISBN 0-8016-2121-8

The new edition of Jeppesen's ADVANCED SPORT DIVER MANUAL is written by a prominent team of dive experts and edited by Richard Clinchy. An attractive two-color design with full-color sections makes the book visually exciting for readers. The popular format and organization have been retained in this edition. New and expanded topics include:

- More information on computers.
- Special sections on beach diving, night diving, cave diving and mixed gas diving.
- Thoroughly updated information on equipment, safety, and diving techniques reflects current diving standards.
- Package includes Instructor's Guide, Workbook, Dive Table, and Log Book.

A MEDICAL GUIDE TO HAZARDOUS MARINE LIFE
2nd Edition

Paul S. Auerbach   1991   ISBN 0-8016-6322-9

A MEDICAL GUIDE TO HAZARDOUS MARINE LIFE provides both the experienced and novice diver with a handy tool for recognizing and treating hazardous marine bites and exposures. The Divers Alert Network (DAN) and the Professional Association of Dive Instructors (PADI) endorse A MEDICAL GUIDE TO HAZARDOUS MARINE LIFE as a quality and thorough resource. Author Paul Auerbach is recognized internationally as an expert on hazardous marine animals, as well as wilderness and environmental emergencies. Consolidates in a single resource practical advice that the diver would otherwise have to seek through numerous sources.

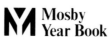

Mosby
Year Book

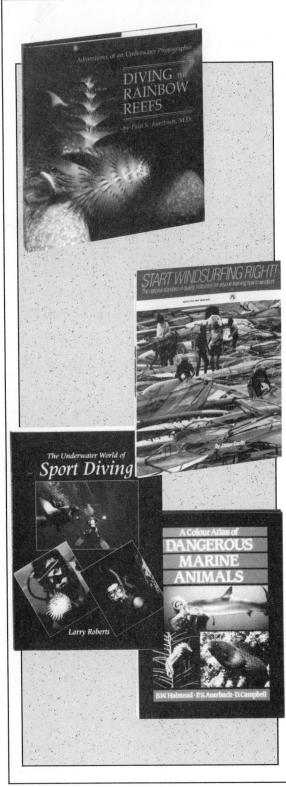
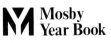